Facing Cancer and the Fear of Death

Facing Cancer and the Fear of Death

A Psychoanalytic Perspective on Treatment

Edited by Norman Straker

ROWMAN & LITTLEFIELD
Lanham • Boulder • New York • London

Published by Rowman & Littlefield
A wholly owned subsidiary of The Rowman & Littlefield Publishing Group, Inc.
4501 Forbes Boulevard, Suite 200, Lanham, Maryland 20706
www.rowman.com

Unit A, Whitacre Mews, 26-34 Stannery Street, London SE11 4AB

British Library Cataloguing in Publication Information Available

Library of Congress Cataloging-in-Publication Data
The hardback edition of this book was previously catalogued by the Library of Congress as follows:

Facing cancer and the fear of death : a psychoanalytic perspective on treatment / edited by Norman Straker.
p.; cm.
Includes bibliographical references and index.
I. Straker, Norman. [DNLM: 1. Neoplasms—psychology. 2. Attitude to Death. 3. Health Personnel—psychology. 4. Psychoanalysis. 5. Survivors—psychology. 6. Terminally Ill—psychology. QZ 200]
616.99'4—dc23
2012044631

ISBN 978-0-7657-0965-3 (cloth : alk. paper)
ISBN 978-1-4422-4299-9 (pbk : alk. paper)
ISBN 978-0-7657-0966-0 (electronic)

Printed in the United States of America

Contents

Acknowledgments

My patients were my greatest teachers and it was a great privilege to have been chosen to share their challenge facing death. Their courage and wisdom is the inspiration for this book. They will never be forgotten. Special acknowledgments should begin with Carolyn Straker, my wife who supported and encouraged me during the entire writing process. She also assisted in the editing and proofreading process.

I am especially grateful to the contributors to the book: Abby Adams-Silvan, John W. Barnhill, Daniel Birger, M. Philip Luber, Molly Maxfield, Alison C. Philips, Patricia Plopa, Tom Pysczynski, Sheldon Solomon, Hillel Swiller, and David P. Yuppa.

I also wish to acknowledge some dear colleagues and friends who provided me with critical and valuable feedback. They include Lowell Rubin, MD, Michael Fleischer, MD, Hillel Swiller, MD, Philip Hahn, Richard M. Gottleieb, MD, and Leon Hoffman, MD. I am especially indebted to my mentor, colleague, and friend for over thirty-five years, Jimmie Holland, MD, Wayne E. Chapman Chair in psycho-oncology at Memorial Sloan-Kettering, who guided me in the study and treatment of the emotional needs of cancer patients and their families. William Breitbart, MD, acting chair of psychiatry and behavioral science at Sloan-Kettering, has also been a great friend and colleague over many decades. Amy King, acquisitions editor of Jason Aronson, was the first to recognize the possibility of this book and I thank her for her foresight. Finally, Stephanie Brooks, assistant editor of production, and Sandi Frank, who is responsible for the index, have been very helpful to me.

Norman Straker, MD

Introduction

Facing Cancer and the Fear of Death:
A Challenge for the Twenty-First Century

Norman Straker, MD

A PSYCHOANALYTIC PERSPECTIVE ON TREATMENTS

The future of health care delivery and our budget deficits are a focus of current national attention. We cannot successfully address these issues until we examine the impact of "death anxiety" on the treatment decisions in the last months of a patient's life. Our society's avoidance of facing death frequently interferes with empowering patients and families on their best options for quality of life when further active treatments are futile. The default position of avoidance creates needless suffering of dying patients, excessive burdens for families, and expenditures of one-third of the Medicare budget in the last year of a patient's life. A total of 20 percent of Americans spend their last days in the intensive care units (ICUs) hooked up to machines that do nothing but isolate the dying person from friends and family (Jacoby, 2011).

The labeling of the plan for end-of-life counseling as "Obama's death panels" exemplifies how easily death anxiety is manipulated for political purpose. Our society is unrealistic and unwilling to accept the limits of our doctors' ability to cure diseases and is quick to avoid any discussions that require us to face death. At the same time, most of our doctors are greatly discomforted by their "failure" to cure their patients and face death themselves. Many avoid the discomfort of discussions about end-of-life care and palliation, collude with their patient's unrealistic hope for cure, and continue futile treatments. Our sophisticated technology can now prolong life almost indefinitely, regardless of quality, and well beyond the point where any recovery can occur. This practice is far too frequent, causes unnecessary suffering for dying patients and excessive trauma for families, and is a waste of our health care resources that could be allocated to better purposes.

One of the goals of this book is to help doctors, psychoanalysts, mental health professionals, patients, their families, hospital administrators, and policy makers face death with less anxiety and apprehension. The task of helping doctors face death more rationally begins with medical student selection, education, and continuing medical education (CME) post-graduate courses on end-of-life care. I think the recommendation for "apportioning more weight in the admissions decisions to characteristics of (medical student) applicants in the interpersonal domains of medicine" by the American Medical Association (AMA) is a step in the right direction. We also need to address the culture of medical education that continues to emphasize "see one, do one, and teach one." This pressure intentionally leaves no room for the personal feelings of the young student learning to accept the responsibility for the health and life of patients. Typical feelings such as fear, sadness, grief, guilt, and shame have always been considered off-limits in the medical setting. If these feelings are expressed, they have been thought of as indications of a lack of capacity to function as a doctor. This suppression of emotion leads to progressive distancing, dissociation, and a loss of empathy with patients, particularly dying patients. We now know that doctors frequently exposed to death tend to suppress their feelings, dissociate, and are vulnerable to posttraumatic stress disorder (PTSD), grief, anxiety, and depression. These symptoms perpetuate their avoidance of facing death and increase false hopes and futile care. These maladaptive coping strategies and burnout are described in the chapters that follow: a memoir by a psycho-oncology fellow, case reports by psychoanalysts of dying patients who were receiving futile treatments by oncologists, and finally, cases of wounded oncologists treated by the author.

Individual case reports in this book by psychoanalysts also describe their discomfort in treating dying patients. Their acknowledgement of countertransference feelings, evoked by facing death with a patient, are processed rather than suppressed or denied. This healthy response to overwhelming feelings suggests a more adaptable coping strategy for medical schools and post-graduate education. Changing how doctors deal with death requires changing how doctors in training and doctors in practice are expected to react to suffering, death, and loss. If we encourage and support them to accept and express their feelings to faculty and colleagues, we will help them to stay connected to their patients rather than dissociating and distancing. This recommendation for a change in approach goes beyond the teaching of "whole person care," which emphasizes training for the relief of suffering and healing as a complement to the disease focus of biomedicine (Hutchinson, Mount, & Kearney, 2011). In addition, oncology and psycho-oncology fellows and residents in the hospital should have group support and perhaps a mandatory debriefing following the death of one their patients. Referrals to a psychoanalyst for a brief therapy might be considered more routinely. Communication skills training, which is now taught, is not enough.

Dr. Yuppa's memoir (chapter 2) and Dr. Luber's case presentation (chapter 11) highlight the impact of an oncologist denying imminent death, continuing futile care, and the resulting unnecessary suffering of patients, families, and doctors. These case reports suggest that reaching a rational decision to discontinue active treatments and initiate discussions on the need for palliative care for some individual oncologists may be so complex that new hospital committees should be established to evaluate the appropriateness of further care. At the same time, mental health professionals should be consulted when unconscious conflicts result in misunderstandings between patients, family members, and doctors about future treatment goals. Ultimately, the goal is for more palliative care at the end of life with less suffering for patients, families, and doctors.

A second but less frequent consequence of death anxiety is blunt communication by the oncologist about survival time, delivered in an offhanded manner with no time for discussion. I have had several referrals of patients who were told abruptly, "You have three months to live, there is nothing that can be done." Greater ease with facing death should result in more relaxed discussions with the patient about the opportunity for palliative or hospice care and limit the psychological trauma of being given a death sentence.

Another goal of this book is to help psychoanalysts be more aware of death anxiety, their own fear of death, and be at greater ease with facing death with their patients. Sigmund Freud's followers have denied the importance of fear of death. This view has resulted in a tendency of psychoanalysts to fail to recognize death anxiety in their clinical work, and relatively few have chosen to treat dying patients. I am hopeful that this book will encourage psychoanalysts to be more open to treating patients with cancer and those facing death.

Reports of treatments of dying patients by psychoanalysts are very limited in psychoanalytic literature. Most psychoanalytic case reports have been rejected by mainstream journals because they do not fit the classical analytic paradigm. Published case reports of dying patients appear in other journals or books. I will review both types: patients treated with minimal modification of orthodox technique and others who were treated with a more flexible approach (see chapter 6).

My approach recognizes that facing cancer and death is a unique life crisis. I view it as special challenge that needs to have a primary focus in the "here and now." Death anxiety cannot be denied indefinitely, nor can it be analyzed away. It is not the same as analyzing neurotic conflicts or transfer-

ences. It requires an approach that is, above all, more flexible than an orthodox approach.

An existential approach is essential to the treatment of patients facing
death. A chapter in this book, "Finding Meaning in Death: Terror Management among the Terminally Ill" (Maxfield, Pyszczynski, & Solomon), describes how terminally ill patients best cope using a terror management approach.

Case reports by both hospital-based and office-based psychoanalysts illustrate how a psychoanalytically trained therapist can lessen the sufferings
of patients facing death and can be a catalyst for emotional growth and
creativity at the end of life. Special emphasis is placed on transference and
countertransference issues. Detailed accounts of what the analysts are feeling
and thinking as they treat their patients is an important feature.

In chapter 12, a psychoanalyst candidate reports on the impact of her
diagnosis of breast cancer on her training analysis. The reader is informed
about the effectiveness of her psychoanalytic treatment on her ability to cope
with facing cancer and death while continuing to treat her patients. The
analyst also describes the impact of her cancer diagnosis on her patients and
her management of their emotional reactions. She also reviews the literature
on how analysts manage their patients when they are ill.

In an effort to give the reader a very intimate experience with facing
death, I have asked two senior psychoanalytic colleagues of mine to write
about their personal journeys with facing cancer and death (chapter 3). Miraculously, both were saved and have agreed to educate us about being at the
edge where death seemed imminent and was accepted. Perhaps most surpris-
ing is the fact that once the fear of death was confronted directly it became
less toxic and frightening and was accepted somewhat peacefully. Loving
family members, friends, and caring staff caretakers allowed for a sense of
calm, creativity, emotional growth, and integration. The founder of the palliative care movement first described this phenomenon as "patients can die
healed" (Hutchinson, Mount, & Kearney, 2011).

Finally, we ask that politicians and policy makers show more courage and
not hide from end-of-life issues. This is one of the major challenges of the
twenty-first century. It requires a multidisciplinary approach that includes
doctors, ethicists, psycho-oncologists, psychoanalysts, lawyers, clergy, rep-
resentatives of insurance companies, and policy makers. If we fail to act, we
will live to see rationing in all of medical care. That will be a great disservice
to all our citizens, but especially to those who could have been restored to a
life with quality but were subject to rationing and denied care.

REFERENCES

Hutchinson, T. A., Mount, B. M., & Kearney, M. (2011). The healing journey. In T. A. Hutchinson (Ed.), *Whole person care: A new paradigm for the 21st century.* Quebec: Springer.

Jacoby, S. (2011). *Never say die: The myth and marketing of old age.* New York: Pantheon Books.

I

Medical Section

Chapter One

The Avoidance of Facing Death

Its Consequences to Our Patients, Families,
Medical Students, and Young Physicians

Norman Straker, MD

WHERE WE ARE NOW

When the bill for affordable health care was found to include a fee for "end-of-life counseling," it was quickly described by the opposition as a fee for "death panels to pull the plug on Grandma." Once again, our avoidance of facing death and a lack of courage by any constituency to pursue a reasonable discourse on this issue has resulted in a lost opportunity to deal with one of the most important challenges of our time. The dying patient would be denied the opportunity for financial reimbursement for mandated counseling about end-of-life decisions. The emotional burden on the dying patients and their families, as well the excessive expenditures at the end of life, were considered to be less problematic than facing death honestly in the public arena. The time should be near when we will become less prone to denial and more aware of what William James has termed "the worm at the core of human existence": our fear of death (James, 1958 [1902]). This book is an effort in that direction. Doctors, psychoanalysts, academics, philosophers, and politicians need to step forward to begin the needed dialogue. Death needs to be detoxified and faced realistically.

The press has been in the forefront recently and has begun to acknowledge the discomfort we all have in facing death. There have been articles on the doctors' discomfort with informing patients and family members that their heroic measures are not going to be productive toward any kind of quality of life. Several articles noted that the word "death" is even avoided on cancer hospital wards (*New York Times*: Brody, 2012; Grady, 2010; Ofri, 2011; *New Yorker*: Gwande, 2010). A recent cover story of *New York Magazine* (May 28, 2012) titled, "Mom, I Love You. I Also Wish You Were Dead. And I Expect You Do, Too" is to the point. This is a son's story of his elderly mother's repetitive medical interventions that repeatedly tried to save her from dying but at enormous costs and for no good purpose. Each medical intervention caused great suffering and a downward spiral of mental functioning. Like so many stories of this kind, futile care can only be avoided with specific advance directives or realistic discussions about the benefits of any new medical intervention.

"The Crushing Cost of Medical Care" (Adamy & McGinty, *Wall Street Journal*, July 7–9, 2012) reviews the $2.1 million cost for hospital care of a forty-one-year-old man before he died in less than one year. The attending cardiologist at Johns Hopkins is quoted as saying "there is an assumption on everyone's part that if heroic things need to be done we are going to do them." In his last year of life, the patient had a defibrillator and heart pump implanted, two separate heart transplants, and multiple infectious complications requiring removal of a gangrenous gall bladder and an above-knee amputation. Kidney and respiratory failure led to dialysis and mechanical ventilation. At this point, because the patient was unable to speak, the critical care specialist approached the patient's father to tell him that he didn't think his son would make it. The father demanded they press forward. The ethics committee then contacted the family in response to the nurse's "moral distress" about caring for a patient with overwhelming pain and suffering. The parents demanded a transfer out of the unit if the nurses could not handle the care. An overwhelming sepsis was the incident that finally convinced the father to take his son off the machines and let him die.

The report is rich with the emotional conflicts involved in the care of this dying patient: doctors, specialists, surgeons, parents, patient, nurses, ethics committees, insurance companies, government agencies. It is noteworthy that there is no mental health consultant involved in this case, as the core issues here involve sorting out the unconscious motivations of each of the players. Perhaps a mental health intervention earlier in the process would have led to less suffering and less wasted resources.

LONG-TERM ACUTE CARE

In the 1990s Congress created a new separate reimbursement under Medicare for long-term acute care (LTAC). A new practice culture emerged that allowed for any patient who could not be weaned from the ventilator within fourteen days to be transferred to LTAC for long-term mechanical ventilation. Since that time, the number of LTAC facilities has increased from 192 to 408 between 1997 to 2006 with a corresponding increase in Medicare payments from \$484 million to \$1.325 billion (Kahn et al., 2010) The Medicare program in 2007 instituted a moratorium on new LTAC hospitals as a result of the rapid growth. It is now clear that rationing on a financial basis will occur if we do not either address or prioritize individual patient entitlement for extended care and end-of-life care decision making. It is important to see where we are in advance directives and preparing for such eventualities. Did patients have an opportunity to decide whether they wanted LTAC? It's not likely given the low percent of the population with advance directives.

WHERE WE ARE: ADVANCE DIRECTIVES, PATIENTS, AND DOCTORS AS PATIENTS

Only 30 percent of Americans have advance directives while most Americans say they want to have some control over how they die (Pew Research Center Report, 2007). The default medical position in cancer, heart disease, and strokes is to keep fighting with all the resources of modern medicine. The first essential requirement of the good ending that nine out of ten Americans say they want is a willingness to face death, yet only two out of ten actually have that conversation (Jacoby, 2011).

A recent study describes the failure of the majority of physicians to comply with the guidelines that recommend end-of-life care discussions with cancer patients who have a life expectancy of less than a year. In the study of more than two thousand patients with newly diagnosed stage IV lung or colorectal cancer, nearly half of lung cancer patients and 22 percent of the colorectal cancer patients died without any discussion at all (Mack et al., 2012).

A recent study reported on the prevalence and predictors of advance directives in patients with congestive heart failure living in Olmsted County, Minnesota. Investigators enrolled 608 of 827 consecutive patients with incident or previously diagnosed heart failure who were seen in a hospital or clinic. Only 41 percent had advance directives, 90 percent of which appointed a surrogate decision maker. A minority of advance directives expressed preferences about resuscitation (41 percent), mechanical ventilation (39 percent), or dialysis (10 percent). Older age, malignancy, and renal dysfunction were predictors of having an advance directive. Compared with patients who were without an advance directive, those with an advance directive had less mechanical ventilation in the last month before death (Dunlay, Swetz, Mueller, & Roger, 2012).

Clearly it is not easy for doctors to talk about or face death. The reasons why include: they are afraid to upset their patients, they are reluctant to face the emotional responses of the patients and family, they want to preserve an optimistic outlook, they fear failure, they may also be in denial themselves, and finally, they want the patients to continue to love them and this relationship changes once death is discussed. The family also plays a role in this problem. Relatives often tend to irrationally opt for the idea that everything that can be done should be done in an effort to avoid guilty feelings. Some doctors even fear litigation. When rounding with doctors, it has been my experience that we tended to most often visit the dying patients last, spent the least amount of time talking to them, and, furthermore, stood at the door entrance rather than enter the room when talking with them. Both are reluctant to initiate any discussion about death, preferring instead to talk about interventions that distract from the inevitable. Doctors even avoid the word "death" when they talk to each other on the wards. Instead they use euphemisms.

There are two bad outcomes that result from the discomfort that doctors have with talking about death. The discussion might be totally avoided or delayed or it may be carried out in a very hurried fashion. If the discussion is delayed, the patients continue in costly, painful, futile treatment and the opportunity for planning for palliation or hospice is missed. If, on the other hand, the communication is hurried, blunt, and definitive, without time for discussion, the patients are psychologically traumatized and feel as if they have been given a death sentence. I will illustrate several examples I have treated where the patients and family responded as if they were given the date when they expected to die, not unlike a date for delivery of a baby.

"Why Doctors Die Differently" appeared in the *Wall Street Journal* (Ofri, February 25, 2012) as an interesting op-ed piece. In a 2003 survey of 765 doctors, Joseph J. Gallo reported that 64 percent had advance directives versus 20 percent for the general population. Almost all doctors have seen futile care being performed on people, especially in the ICU and in patients with terminal disease. Doctors do not want someone breaking their ribs by performing cardiopulmonary resuscitation (CPR) at the end of their life. A study of more than 95,000 cases of CPR found that only 8 percent of patients survived for more than a month and only 3 percent were able to live a normal life (Yasunuga et al. 2010). Therefore, they are more inclined to advance directives. A study by Susan Diem of CPR performed on TV showed a 75 percent success rate with 67 percent of TV cases going home for a normal life. The general public gets their information mostly from TV; the doctors have a more realistic view.

Doctors administer a great deal of medical care that they would not want for themselves. This is, of course, a very provocative finding and raises lots of questions as to why. Our culture overpromises what is possible and this is reflected in the unrealistic expectations of the physician and its impact on the doctor patient relationship. On the patient's side, there is misinformation, unrealistic expectations, and a denial of death. On the doctor's side, an ena-bling role may be the result in an effort to avoid the discomfort of talking about death and intense emotions such as sadness, anger, etc., and wishing to fulfill the patient and family's omnipotent wishes. It is clear that the public deserves more education and fees for end-of-life counseling so that there is an opportunity for patients to make informed choices.

AVOIDANCE OF DEATH IN MEDICAL SCHOOL CONTINUES

I rely on my own experience and the experience of my son who is a recent medical school graduate. It is also my impression, based on my experience teaching residents and fellows for many years, including the psycho-oncolo-gy fellow who wrote his memoir for this book, that little, if anything, has changed in the training of medical students in regard to the stress of facing death. I remember my first day of medical school as a young medical student with horror. We were casually introduced to our cadavers without any prep-aration or discussion. My first cut into the cadaver was the first of many traumatic experiences in medical school that changed me. I was being pre-pared psychologically to be an objective doctor. Looking back on this experi-ence as a psychoanalyst, I now believe that this frightening experience with no preparation began the unconscious psychological defensive split between the patient and me. Cadavers, our first patients, were made very distinct from us, the healthy "immortal medical students." Our defense against death, "our specialness," was being established through distancing, intellectualization, splitting, and dissociation. My psychoanalytic training analysis served as an antidote to this dissociative process and was responsible for my rediscover-ing my empathy toward suffering patients.

A recent survey of the prevalence of burnout, stress, depression, and the use of supports by medical students at one school supports my view that the culture in medical school is as stressful now as when I was a medical student (Chang et al., 2012). The results showed that 55 percent scored in the high burnout range, and 60 percent showed significant depressive symptoms using a variety of measuring instruments. The most helpful coping strategies were social supports from peers and faculty, counseling services, and extracurricu-lar activities.

INTERNSHIP: MY FIRST PATIENT DIES

This life experience was one of many that helped shape my unconscious interest in teaching medical students, doctors, psychoanalysts, and psychi-atrists to be more comfortable in facing and discussing death. While this experience proved to be somewhat traumatic for me, it was not disruptive and, in fact, led me to a desire for greater mastery rather than avoidance.

Within weeks of starting my internship I was confronted alone with a young woman who died within hours of admission, another traumatic experience. Early one evening, when all the senior staff had gone home, an asymptomatic eighteen-year-old woman with tiny red spots on her legs was sent to my floor for diagnosis and treatment. Emergency blood studies revealed acute leukemia and a very low platelet count. Within hours the patient who had been well on admission was having grand mal seizures from a brain hemorrhage. I treated her seizures with intravenous Valium, worrying all the while that I might give her an overdose and cause her death while trying to control her convulsions. After she died, it was then my responsibility to attempt to console her parents and try to help them cope with this overwhelming tragedy. I did this with great difficulty, never having been trained to deal with such an eventuality. I was fortunate to have some innate skills and a family that was able to try to accept this tragedy and not become enraged at me. The next morning, when the medical staff returned to the hospital, my recollection was that when I described this case on morning rounds, it was treated routinely without any comment or consolation. Looking back, I was extremely fortunate that the response of the patient's family was accepting, understanding, and not condemning.

THE CULTURE OF A CANCER HOSPITAL CONSTRUCTED TO AVOID DEATH AT THE TOP AND ITS IMPACT ON ONCOLOGY RESIDENTS FELLOWS AND FELLOWS IN PSYCHO-ONCOLOGY

It is my impression that most of the oncology departments in hospitals are set up so that the senior faculty at the top of the hierarchy are shielded from many of the daily issues of the hospitalized cancer patients: the pain, anguish, suffering, anxiety, depression, and demoralization. The faculty can often avoid the daily bedside rounds with the patient and family by rounding with fellows and residents separately where they decide on the treatment regimen and access the progress of the treatments. The patients are often unable to identify any one senior doctor as their own because of the scheduling of physicians, on service or off service, research, or travel commitments for lectures of conferences. The daily experience of treating patients is allocated to the rotating residents and fellows on the service. They witness the suffering of cancer patients and their families at eye level and confront life and death emergencies. They quickly become highly competent in the actual management of the illness component. At the same time, they develop coping strategies to insulate themselves from the emotional helplessness of witnessing death and suffering. These coping mechanisms include avoidance, dissociation, intellectualization, and compartmentalization. This process is aided by the availability of psycho-oncologists or psychiatrists who readily appear when there is a perceived psychological issue. If a patient or family member demonstrates any psychological discomfort or is upset, regardless of the cause, the psycho-oncologist is called.

The primary trauma for the oncology residents and fellows is their inability to conquer death and the consequence to them of losing their patients. The psycho-oncology fellows with whom I have worked play a different role and their suffering is different. They are traumatized by witnessing the suffering of their patients and at times feel helpless, unable to influence the outcome of either the illness or the continuation of toxic futile treatments. They also grieve for the loss of patients to whom they have become attached. This book will describe the psychoanalytic therapy of an oncology fellow, and a memoir by a psycho-oncology fellow will provide a closer look at life in the trenches in a cancer hospital.

A study devoted to explore and identify the impact of loss and grief on oncologists and its impact on their personal and professional lives (Granek et al., 2012) is central to my thesis. Interviews of twenty oncologists regarding their experiences related to loss of their patients were recorded and transcribed. The data was subject to analysis and the following results were reported. Oncologists reported sadness, crying, and loss of sleep. These are frequent symptoms of grief. A unique finding was related to the sense of responsibility over patients' lives resulting in feelings of powerlessness, self-doubt, guilt, and failure. The use of "denial" and "dissociation" words chosen by the oncologists allowed them to cope by compartmentalizing their patient experiences. Remaining emotionally distant to their patients was acknowledged as a method to avoid the pain of loss, with greater distance from the patient and family as the death was approaching. However, the compartmentalization was often an unsuccessful defense and resulted in "grief spillover"—that is, grieving at home and distraction at work. The article's final comment is particularly relevant:

> For oncologists, patient loss was a unique affective experience that had a smoke-like quality. Like smoke, this grief was intangible and invisible. Nonetheless, it was pervasive, sticking to the physicians' clothes when they went home after work and slipping under the doors between patient rooms. Of greatest significance to our health care system is that some of the oncologists' reactions to grief reported in our study (altered treatment decisions, mental distraction, emotional and physical withdrawal from patients) suggest that the failure of oncologists to deal appropriately with grief from patient loss may negatively affect not only oncologists, but also patients and their families. One way to begin to ameliorate these negative effects would be to provide education to oncologists on how to manage difficult emotions such as grief. Starting at the residency stage and throughout their careers, oncologists need to recog-

nize that grief is a sensitive topic that can produce shame and embarrassment for the mourner.

TREATMENT OF ONCOLOGISTS

I was referred an oncology fellow who had been deeply depressed for more than a year. Although he had no conscious awareness that he was depressed, he was described as not being like himself for about one year despite being able to continue to work. He did, however, describe symptoms of anxiety especially before night call or clinic, a general level of tiredness, a lack of interest in socializing, a loss of interest in physical fitness, weight gain, and a diminished sexual desire. He had also noticed that he had significantly increased his alcohol consumption.

He dated the onset of his symptoms to the death of one his patients approximately his age about a year ago. His patient had been terminally ill and in a lot of pain. As his patient began to experience respiratory distress, the oncology fellow spoke with his patient about the option for a tracheotomy. This procedure would keep the patient alive, but he would be unconscious and it would interfere with his last hours with his family. The patient chose to decline the procedure. He died before the family had reached a stage of acceptance of his death. The patient's father and brother screamed angrily immediately after his death, "You let him die, you could have saved him," and the mother sobbed almost continuously.

The oncology fellow suffered frequent night terrors after this event. He would awaken from his sleep to the screams of the patient's family. Sharing his experience with me, as well as discussing his feelings of survivor guilt, was helpful. We began a weekly psychotherapy. He was also treated with Buprioprion for depression. During these visits he acknowledged that he periodically reviewed the care he gave to other children who died, questioning whether everything that could have been done was done. His sessions allowed him to grieve and review his decisions and face the survivor guilt associated with his not dying. He also acknowledged that before he had been depressed he had enjoyed a great sense of camaraderie, gallows humor, and many happy hours spent with his fellow cancer specialists. However, they never shared the details of the most troublesome conflicts that resulted from their attending dying patients.

ATTENDING ONCOLOGISTS

Dr. X consulted me after a vivid confrontation with the impact of his work on his personal life. He had been a dedicated oncologist for more than twenty years. He was a happily married man with three children. He realized that something was wrong after his wife reported to him that she was in a car with her three children when a truck hit them. The car was totaled, his children and his wife miraculously were unhurt, and "I felt nothing."

We agreed to a weekly psychotherapy. The challenge I faced was to help him reconnect with his feeling experiences. We began with a review of the loss of some of his early patients. He had never mourned his losses, but instead dissociated. He compartmentalized his work. He had thought that this was the best method of being able to do his work. However, he did so without experiencing the music in his life. A detailed review of many of his relationships with his patients permitted him to accept his sadness and begin grieving. His expression of feelings was initially confined to the sessions and gradually extended to home and work. I tried to encourage him to speak about his feelings to colleagues and his wife, which he had previously not done. He found this to be more adaptive than managing everything himself.

I also recollect treating another oncologist, who also suffered from intense survivor guilt. He was referred to me in the very last days of his wife's illness. She was terminally ill with stage IV breast cancer. She was, unfortunately, suffering from a great deal of pain near the end of her life, but opted to remain at home. This illness occurred before the era of home hospice, so in order to stay at home the husband agreed to administer the IM Demerol as routinely prescribed. After she stopped breathing he was racked with guilt, and when he confessed to me that he might have caused her death, we reviewed together what doses he had given in the last twenty-four hours. Although the doses he administered were standard, when we first talked he had been unable to remember the usual doses and was sure he caused her death. I assured him that he had not and that he would soon remember the standard doses but that he needed to accept that he was suffering from survivor guilt. In this case, it was very clear that he had been in great psychological pain watching his wife in her last days. As in most situations, he was wishing for the horrible ordeal to be over, and when it was he was confused as to whether he had mistakenly caused the wished-for end to actually happen.

REFERENCES

Adamy, J., & McGinty, T. (2012, July 7–9). The crushing cost of medical care. *Wall Street Journal*, online: wsj.com.

Brody, H. M. D., PhD. (2010). Medicine's ethical responsibility for health care reform—The top five list. *New England Journal of Medicine, 362*, 283–285.

———. (2012). From an ethics of rationing to an ethics of waste avoidance. *New England Journal of Medicine, 366*, 1949–1951.

Brody, J. (2010, March 15). When hope is your only peaceful ending. *The New York Times.*

———. (2012, May 28). When costly medical care just adds to the pain, personal health. *The New York Times.*

———. (2012, May 29). Trimming a bloated health care system. *The New York Times.*

Chang, E. D., Eddins-Folensbee, E., & Coverdale, J. (2012). Survey of the prevalence of burnout, stress, depression, and the use of supports by medical students at one school. *Academic Psychiatry, 36*(3), 177–182. DOI: 10.1176/appi.ap.11040079.

Dunlay, S. M., Swetz, K. M., Mueller, P. S., & Roger, V. L. (2012). Advance directives in community patients with heart failure. *Circulation: Cardiovascular Quality and Outcomes, 5*, 283.

Grady, D. (2010, January 11). Facing end of life talks, doctors choose to wait. *The New York Times*.

Granek, L. (2012, May 27). When doctors grieve. *The New York Times*, 12.

Granek, L., PhD; R. Tozer, MD; P. Mazzotta, MD, CCFP, MSc; A. Ramjaun, BHSc; & M. Krzyzanowska, MD, MPH. (2012). Nature and impact of grief over patient loss on oncologists' personal and professional lives. *Archives of Internal Medicine*, 1–3. DOI: 10.1001/archinternmed.2012.1426.

Gwande, A. (2010, July 20). Letting go. *The New Yorker*.

Jacoby, S. (2011). *Never say die: The myth and marketing of the new old age*. New York: Pantheon.

James, W. (1958 [1902]). *Varieties of religious experience: A study in human nature*. New York: Mentor Edition.

Kahn, J. M., Benson, N. M., Appleby, D., Carson, S. S., & Jwashyna, T. J. (2010). Long-term acute care hospital utilization after critical illness. *Journal of the American Medical Association, 303*, 2253–2259.

Keating, N., Landrum, M. K., Roger, S. O., Jr., Baum, S. K., Virnig, B. A., Huskamp, H. A. et al. (2010). Physician factors associated with discussions about the end of life care. *Cancer*, 1–10.

Mack, J. W., Cronin, A., Tabach, N., Huskamp, H. A., Keating, N. L., Malin, J. L. et al. (2012). End of life care discussions among patients with advanced cancer: A cohort study. *Annals of Internal Medicine*, 156–204.

Ofri, D. (2011, May 26). Doctors and the 'd' word. *The New York Times*.

———. (2012, February 25). Why doctors die differently. *Wall Street Journal*.

Rie, M. A. (2012). Mechanical ventilation: Costs, consequences, and accountability for access disparities. *Critical Care Medicine, 40*(4), 1351–1352.

Wolff, M. (2012, May 28). Mom, I love you. I also wish you were dead. And I expect you do, too. *New York Magazine*.

Yasunuga, H., et al. (2010). Collaborative effects of bystander-initiated cardiopulmonary resuscitation and pre-hospital advance cardiac life support by physicians on survival of out-of-hospital cardiac arrest: A nationwide population based observational study. *Critical Care, 14*(6), R199.

Chapter Two

A Fellow's Perspective on Facing Death

David P. Yuppa, MD, with Norman Straker, MD

My goal in this piece is to add a brief memoir of my psycho-oncology fellowship training at Memorial Hospital, which has been the most meaningful experience of my life. Detailed accounts of the patients, families, and staff who forever touched my heart and soul during this period could fill volumes. During that time, I became very aware of some of the shortcomings of the current medical approach to facing death. As a result, I have become very interested in teaching and writing about the subject of death and dying, and I am interested in attempting to affect a cultural shift in how we doctors deal with death. I believe the answer lies in the education of future medical students and graduate medical education. It will be a challenge to significantly alter the way established practitioners tend to avoid talking to their patients about death as they get closer to dying and fail to recommend early palliative care (despite the work of Temel[1] and others). Unfortunately, many doctors believe that palliative care is hospice or comfort care and view it as a defeat or failure. This is not their fault, however; they were simply never taught otherwise.

With few exceptions, I noticed the avoidance of death was being passed down from one generation to the next in my non-psychiatric colleagues. We are taught in medical school that maintaining a safe distance from patients is crucial to the process of objectivity. Indeed, even (and especially) in psychiatry, boundaries and distance are moving targets subject to change with each and every encounter. It seems that somewhere along the way, this objectivity and boundary maintenance has resulted in an avoidance of confronting, talking about, or even mentioning death. The unfortunate result that I have repeatedly observed and will recount in this memoir is the unnecessary aggressive treatment to prolong the lives of people with diseases that are terminal at the time of diagnosis or admission. This practice contributes to the burden of sick patients, caregivers, and families, and adds to the trauma of the doctors themselves. Death is delayed temporarily, but often at the expense of living out one's days with some degree of quality. When death inevitably arrives, health care providers are often filled with feelings of sadness, impotence, and failure. As a result, death is experienced as a trauma or injury. For those who dedicate their lives to treating cancer patients, these traumas are omnipresent and neverending. Without appropriate processing of such emotions, many practitioners become numb or detached. The "baptism by fire" and "see one, do one, teach one" mantras of medical education allow these maladaptive mechanisms to continue. Unfortunately, my experience has shown me that in some physicians, this detachment results in their distancing from the patient and, at times, feels cold.

I believe the trauma of working with dying patients of all ages is experienced more intensely in mental health professionals, especially trainees who provide psychiatric care to cancer patients and their families. Our psychotherapy training teaches us to empathize and forge strong alliances with patients at the worst times of their lives. Our prolonged contact with patients in their times of extreme emotional distress and suffering exposes us to a plethora of emotion. We have come to know the patients for who they were, for what gave their lives meaning. We feel tremendous losses when our patients die. It is painful. To do this work effectively is to engage in great sacrifice. Meaningful empathy and development of close relationships with dying people enhances the sting. We in the psychiatric field do not have the distraction of basic science research and developing experimental treatment protocols. I have witnessed how the hope of being involved in a clinical trial can be a distraction from facing death and sustain patients and their doctors for weeks as their illnesses progressed.

I will now recount several poignant experiences during my fellowship year to illustrate my conclusion that change is necessary. My first exposure to the impact of the denial of an inevitable death was "Amy," a married mother of two children in her early forties who suffered from an aggressive, treatment-resistant sarcoma. Her stage IV sarcoma was classified at the time of diagnosis and was extremely aggressive and resistant to all treatments. Despite this, she had endured extensive surgery and experimental chemotherapy protocols. I first met her in the ICU, as I did many patients in my early months at Memorial. I was asked to make an assessment of whether she was anxious or delirious during an attempted trial of weaning her from a ventilator. I concluded that the causes of her delirium were irreversible; she was terminally ill. I saw her daily for more than three weeks and got to know her family very well. I helped them process their feelings, most of which were anger and immeasurable pain. Eventually, Amy was taken off of the breathing machine and transferred to the wards with a tracheotomy. She was able to experience some brief periods of lucidity and meaningful exchanges with her husband, sister, and parents. As her cancer continued to progress, she was transferred back to intensive care. Her mental status waxed and waned until her ability to have sustained interactions ceased. One of the ongoing dilemmas was whether or not to bring her young children, three and five years old, to visit her prior to discontinuation of life support. The nurses were able to conceal the vast array of catheters, tubes, and other miscellaneous items under a blanket so that the children were not frightened. They brought gifts and pictures to their mother, and after a brief visit, they left smiling. The only tears came from our eyes. Amy died two days later.

This was my first experience of what it was really going to be like doing this work. I experienced the sadness of Amy's life coming to an end, the realization that she would not see her children grow up—no weddings, no birthdays. It was all ending. These poor children had lost their mother before they entered kindergarten. A young husband lost his wife, and her parents lost their daughter. I could not help but wonder if it needn't be this way. She had a health care proxy, but not an advance directive. Why? Was it really necessary to prolong her suffering in the ICU? Amy was a forty-year-old woman with a terminal illness. She had suffered and deteriorated before everyone's eyes. As this process unfolded, I had an epiphany. I realized that the aggressive chemotherapy was doing more harm than good. But her family was given "hope" about possible responses to further anti-neoplastic treatments. There was a conspicuous lack of attention paid to the terminality and futility of the situation. Her husband expressed varying degrees of adaptive denial, but was eventually able to accept the fate of his bride with great courage.

As I reflected on this tragedy, a few things came to mind. Amy was my first patient who died, and I had grown very close to her family. Her death was traumatic for me. I discussed my feelings and experiences with my volunteer faculty mentor. I was able to process everything with him and he proved to be invaluable to me during my year of training. Beyond that, I found myself on an island. Our full-time faculty were available to me and gave of their time during rounds, but the fellows were left to deal with these kinds of traumas on their own. We had each other, but we needed more.

The second patient I think about is "Larry." I'm not sure if there will ever be another patient who will be able to brand my heart as Larry did. Larry was in his early sixties, married, and the father of two young adult children. He was suffering from a gastrointestinal cancer that had metastasized to his brain. I first met Larry during an admission for altered mental status that lasted ten weeks. The unique aspect of Larry's illness was that his cancer was stable and he was otherwise healthy. The location of his brain lesion/resection produced a chronic cognitive impairment that required twenty-four-hour nursing. When his behavioral symptoms were finally under control, the recommendation was made to transfer him to an inpatient hospice. Shortly after he arrived, I received a frantic call from his wife. She was in tears and screaming, "They're telling me Larry is dying!" I knew something was wrong because his general health was fairly good and his cancer was stable. I learned that there had been no meaningful transfer of pertinent information about the unique nature of his illness, and the hospice staff assumed that this cognitive impairment and restlessness was a manifestation of terminal delirium. Larry was placed on a sedative infusion by mistake and had been bedridden for two days. I suspected that he had likely suffered aspiration pneumonia. I convinced the medical director to obtain an x-ray to confirm. Larry was treated with antibiotics and then transferred out of the hospital. I had saved the life of one of my most treasured patients from one hundred miles away. When I hung up the phone I cried. I could not wait to tell my colleagues about this during the following day's case conference.

While relating the events of the previous night I became very emotional. My tale of woe didn't seem to arouse the response I had hoped. Most of the faculty were familiar with this patient. When I explained what had happened and that I had saved his life, I received a "nice job." I was, again, experiencing a trauma on an island. Everyone knew how special this patient and his family were to me. Fortunately, my colleagues were very supportive. So too was my volunteer faculty supervisor. Otherwise, I felt largely invalidated and unsupported.

Another distressing case for me was "Jack." Jack was a prominent retired attorney in his seventies who was suffering from metastatic prostate cancer. I was asked to see him to evaluate a depressive diagnosis. As I entered his room, his lovely wife, who was tending to him at the bedside, greeted me. I also met his accomplished children and saw pictures of the extended family. He was a proud patriarch. It became obvious very quickly that Jack was suffering from hypoactive delirium: a confusional state often mistaken for depression. His level of arousal and activity was underactive and sluggish. I was soon troubled to learn that his oncologist had scheduled chemotherapy for the following day and that the family was optimistic that this would help improve his condition. I spoke with the family, explaining that although their father might appear depressed, he was in fact delirious. We needed to look for the cause. One of the children then mentioned to me that the house staff had recommended hospice, in contrast to the primary oncologist who had planned for chemotherapy the following day. It became clear after a review of his chart that the patient was in the early stages of multi-system organ failure. His liver and kidneys were beginning to shut down, and he was dying. Despite this, the primary oncologist, who was in charge, planned for an ongoing chemotherapy regimen. The patient died the following morning.

"Kimberly" was one of the last patients I worked with during the year, and my reaction to her treatment reflected my frustration and my state of early burnout. She was a lovely young woman in her thirties suffering from a stage IV cholangiocarcinoma. Psychiatry was asked to provide a consultation by the medical oncology service team. They were not comfortable with the level of aggressive treatment she was being given, but they had little influence on the overall management. She had lost more than fifty pounds and was severely cachectic. She suffered from chronic nausea, pain, and failure to thrive. Her oncologist had advanced her chemotherapy regimen even in her very weakened condition. I attempted to engage her in psychotherapy and made pharmacologic recommendations for the treatment of her poor appetite, nausea, anxiety, and insomnia. Her oncologist was known for his aggressive approach and "never giving up" on patients.

I learned from Kimberly's chart and from speaking with her that she never did respond well to any of her treatment regimens. Ten days before she died she was advanced to a more toxic regimen of both systemic and intrahepatic chemotherapy. As she wept and spoke of her intense grief over her life, I found myself surprisingly detached. Kimberly was close to me in age, from a nearby town, and recently married (though her honeymoon was cancelled to start chemotherapy). It was the last month of my academic year and the sadness of her situation was so profound that I found myself unable to feel it. Cognitively, I knew it was heart-wrenching, but I did not feel it. Eventually, a "do not resuscitate" (DNR) order was entered, and Kimberly died peacefully in the hospital with her family by her side. When she died, I was relieved that her suffering was over and enraged at the system that allowed this to happen.

As I review my experience, it is obvious to me that death anxiety was pervasive in our cancer hospital and influencing the treatment of our patients. The anxiety of the doctors is dealt with by avoiding thinking about and talking about death. The excessive chemotherapy treatment in the patients that I have reported upon, which are not anomalies, were not only futile but clearly detrimental to the patients and their families. We psycho-oncology fellows repeatedly witnessed a failure to stop toxic treatments and begin palliation because the signs of approaching death were being denied. This only increased and prolonged the patient's suffering and was the direct antithesis of why I became a doctor: to bring comfort to those who suffer. The fellowship was physically and emotionally grueling enough without this additional struggle against the cultural denial of death. There were countless instances in which, as consultants, we felt as if our hands were tied. It was clear that we were helpless witnesses. The damage had already been done.

When discussing the above patients with my faculty, I became frustrated with the politics of the situation. It was apparent that our interventions were on a case-by-case basis and that the institutional philosophy of aggressive treatment at all times was trumping consideration for good end-of-life care in most instances. I never did receive any acceptable explanations for this. I assumed and was assured that all of these doctors who took this aggressive stance did so because they cared for their patients and wanted to save them. They were under pressure from patients and families to produce miracles. At Memorial Hospital, doctors often treat patients who have failed all other therapies and are looking for cures that simply do not exist. Memorial doctors have the reputation of being very aggressive with their treatments and always striving for the cure. I highlight these disparities not to demonize the oncologists, for I do not envy their difficult position. However, I do believe it is incumbent upon us to face death with the grace and dignity that our patients deserve. Our institutional denial is detrimental. Relying on psychiatry, social work, and the palliative care services to primarily tend to patients' hardships and suffering only worsens the problem. A paradigm shift is necessary.

On reflection, I've attempted to make some sense out of what I experienced. In general, it seemed that younger doctors, less removed from training, were slightly more compassionate. They also seemed to care more for the well-being of their team members (i.e., fellows, residents). The logistics of attending physician schedules also created many boundaries and reprieves from direct patient care. Many doctors made rounds on the wards either in two-week blocks or intermittently at their discretion, often without the primary service team. Due to the great importance placed on research, physicians at Memorial and other prominent cancer centers have great responsibilities outside the realm of patient care. They are charged with securing the future of cancer treatments. To that end, an army of attending physician extenders (graduate medical staff, nurse practitioners, and physician assistants) served as the interlocutors between patients and their doctors. They were the point personnel for dealing with the day-to-day management. I cannot help but wonder if this barrier between the doctor, who is the decision maker guiding the treatment plan, and the patient was contributing to this cultural denial of death. How can we expect young doctors to tend to their patients' spiritual and psychosocial needs if they are not exposed to such an approach in their training?

In our department, attending physicians also had many responsibilities to fulfill other than direct patient care and fellow supervision. We service a very busy outpatient clinic, and research is an institutional priority. Many of our faculty members are also often traveling to spread the knowledge of psycho-oncology across the world. The fellows are in charge of the inpatient service and have outpatient clinic duties as well as research expectations. There is no barrier between the fellows and the patients. We are those most at risk for burnout and traumatic reactions. We are exposed to the emotional pain and suffering of dying patients on a daily basis with little reprieve. As days turned into weeks and weeks into months, the effect that this work was having on all of us became very clear. The tremendous physical and emotional load placed on caregivers in this environment is extremely conducive to burnout, PTSD, anxiety, depression, substance abuse, and so forth.

The overall message is clear: trainees at all levels need much more emotional support than they were receiving during this traumatic process. Many of our fellows enjoyed support from their volunteer faculty mentors during the year. In the very limited free time available, doing things together outside of the hospital was also helpful. Some suggested that making psychotherapy available or even required would be invaluable. Others have suggested mandatory debriefing following the death of patients. Despite the traumatic hardships, losses, and sacrifices, the ability to do this work is a gift. It is a privilege to enter people's lives when they are most vulnerable and in the greatest need of a doctor. I never could have imagined that a year of medical training would have such a profound impact on my life. In many ways, psycho-oncologists have become a throwback of sorts. We spend a great deal of time with patients, communicate effectively, tend to families, and accompany them on their journeys. We ease suffering, allay fears and anxieties, and help our fellow human beings face death with courage and dignity. There is much work to be done in the realm of teaching the eager young minds of tomorrow how to approach one of life's few certainties. Nevertheless, despite all that we do, I stand in awe of those who I have cared for. They have taught me more than I could have ever imagined, and for that I am forever in their debt.

NOTE

1. "Early Palliative Care for Patients with Metastatic Non-Small Cell Lung Cancer" is an article published in 2010 in the *New England Journal of Medicine* in which Dr. Temel and colleagues at Massachusetts General Hospital demonstrated that patients with advanced lung cancer who received early palliative care lived longer and reported higher quality of life scores when compared to their counterparts receiving anti-neoplastic care only (*New England Journal of Medicine, 363*, 733–742).

Chapter Three

Confronting the Fear of Death

Trying to Detoxify Death: Two Memoirs

Daniel Birger, MD, Hillel Swiller, MD, and Norman Straker, MD

"The physicality of death destroys us; the idea of death saves us. The gift of self-awareness is what makes us human and differentiates from other living organisms, but it comes with the price of recognizing that we are mortal" (Yalom, 2008). This confrontation or "awakening" (Yalom's term) occurs at varying points in the life cycle. It varies in intensity depending on the level of emotional awareness that we will die. The knowledge that we are mortal is mostly denied throughout life and remains unconscious until we are forced to confront this reality. These experiences occur with the death of a parent or the celebration of a significant birthday, usually a decade maker such as forty, fifty, sixty, seventy, eighty years of age, that marks the passage of time. Other occasions for awakening include the making of a will, signing advance directives, and appointing health care proxies. However, these awakenings are usually relatively brief, and we very quickly rationalize away our concerns and become re-invested in our life pursuits. The more we re-engage in our usual activities, especially if they bolster our self-esteem, the better we can deny our death anxiety.

However, if one is given a diagnosis of cancer or if a cancer recurs, the terror of death is real, conscious, and palpable for some time. Anxiety, insomnia, dysphoria, depression, anorexia, self-preoccupation, and suffering and withdrawal are common after the bad news is heard. The challenge of coping with the finality of one's life has now really begun. The anxiety is often modulated if the oncologist's treatment plan offers hope of a remission and cure. A relative calmness can occur in the context of a caring relationship with the oncologist who inspires trust. The transference can be very positive and powerful, as the patient feels very frightened and helpless and wants to view the oncologist as omnipotent. Once treatment begins, anxiety is replaced by hope, and denial returns. Anxiety may return if a serious complication results from the toxicity of the treatment. If that happens, the treatment is now recognized to have side effects that can be lethal. Now each laboratory test brings apprehension of possible new danger. The roller coaster experience of cancer that is well-known begins with the first complication.

When the cancer treatment seems to be going well, the patients endure the side effects and ardors of the treatment without much complaint as the price of being cured. The adaptive patients try to go about their life as best they can with little evidence of the fear of death. Denial is again operative. However, each new scan and magnetic resource imaging (MRI) scan interrupts the calm until the results confirm that there is no new growth and the tumor is shrinking.

Panic returns if the oncologist communicates that the cancer treatment is not effective and there is a recurrence or a failure to arrest tumor growth. Hopefully, options are available and can be discussed. Some of the treatments may bring patients into remission; others are toxic and experimental. The most difficult conversation reveals that there are no more options that will arrest the disease.

This conversation—that a cure can no longer be expected—forces patients to face their death. For purposes of discussion we will separate the fear of dying into two parts; the first is fear of going through the dying process and death itself, and the second is accepting the fact that we will no longer exist—the "dread of no longer being" (Kierkegaard, 1957), "the impossibility of further possibility" (Heidegger, 2008 [1927]). Our fears of dying include the fear of pain, of loss of control, of aloneness, of dependency, of being a burden, of losing our dignity, and the inability to help one's own family. Some people also fear the transition to death and being dead. Most of these fears can be lessened by reassurance from a caring doctor, psychoanalyst, psychiatrist, or palliative or hospice care professional, for example, pain will be controlled, the patient will not be abandoned.

The anxiety about being dead for those who are not religious is best looked at with patients using the three arguments of Epicurus, says Irvin Yalom (Yalom, 2008). The clergy best counsels those who are religious. For those who are not so religiously inclined, the first argument of Epicurus is that if we accept that the soul is mortal and perishes with the body, we have nothing to fear in the afterlife. The second is that death is nothingness to us. If we do not perceive where we are, death is not, and where death is, we are not. The final argument of Epicurus is that our state of not being after death is the same state we were in before we were born.

The second major fear is the fear of personal extinction, the end of our life pursuits, and connections without a future (obliteration, extinction, annihilation). The suffering that results from confronting the end of one's existence is intense. There is a heightened awareness of the impending loss and separation from loved ones and everything that is meaningful to you. Acceptance often initiates a chaotic period. The feeling of finiteness and transiency is intense and this can result in life feeling meaningless. Depression and demoralization can occur. The world seems more precarious; danger initially seems to be everywhere. Heidegger refers to this as "uncanniness": the experience of not being at home in the world (Heidegger, 2008 [1927], 223). This imminent reality often brings the patient to the psychoanalyst, psychiatrist, or the clergy.

"Whole person care," a derivative of the palliative care movement, aims for healing in these moments. Healing comes from the acceptance of a change, that cure is no longer possible, and a redirection of hopes and goals to those that are achievable. It is believed to occur through a healing connection from caring caretakers (Hutchinson, Mount, & Kearney, 2011). These ideas have an earlier history in the observations of some of our greatest authors. Personal change after confronting death is a theme, for example, Tolstoy's *War and Peace* (1931), *The Death of Ivan Ilyich* (1960), and the well-known transformation of Ebenezer Scrooge. The recognition of death's nearness creates a sense of poignancy to life, provides a radial shift in life perspective, and can change one's focus to a more authentic mode away from the diversions of everyday life. Heidegger, in 1927's *Being and Time*, notes that the awareness of our own personal death acts to shift our focus to a higher level of existence, from a state of forgetfulness of being (inauthentic) to a state of mindfulness of being (authentic). In the first state, one lives in the world of things and immerses oneself in everyday diversions of life. In the state of mindfulness, one marvels not about the way things are but that they are "in awe of being" (Heidegger, 1927 [2008]).

This awakening experience and the challenge it represents is the impetus for a productive and rewarding psychoanalytic psychotherapy. I have noted that some patients with a lifelong cancer phobia are no longer afraid; in fact, to some degree, many neurotic symptoms disappear. Patients can be encouraged to live more in the now, taking in all that life offers to them in spite of whatever limitations they have. In this vein, an acceptance of mortality can be very liberating, a special time in which the preciousness of life and time is most cherished. Many patients rearrange their life priorities by trivializing life's trivia rather than succumbing to despair. Among the changes that people make are the following: they communicate more deeply with those they love, appreciate nature more fully, are more willing to take risks, are less concerned with rejection, are more eager to seize the day and live in the now. People facing death seem to feel more deeply, are more compassionate, want connection with others, and are eager to teach about their journey. Dr. Daniel Birger's memoir is an excellent example. Those who have mourned their sense of immortality have accepted death and they have reached an integrated state of being grateful for the time they have remaining and using it as best they can. "Count your blessings" is a state of gratitude for the countless givens of existence. This is a predominant theme in Dr. Hillel Swiller's memoir.

This intense connection described in *Whole Person Care* (Hutchinson, Mount, & Kearney, 2011) is the result of the patient's intense needs for security and the availability of caring, humane caregivers at the end of life. This dynamic is especially clear in the description by Daniel Birger, MD, a psychoanalyst who was facing death in the bone marrow transplant unit. He felt loved by family and friends and was intensely in love with many members of the staff. Under those conditions, he found the inner resources to grow and reach a new sense of integrity and wholeness that was different than his status quo. He also recounts the new psychological growth that occurred when his awareness that he would die was most keen. He reviewed his life in great detail, highlighting his abilities to overcome adversity at other times in his life. He conducted a self-analysis. He concluded that he was satisfied that he was proud of the life he had led and was ready to die. He was miraculously saved and we are the richer for his memoir. Dr. Hillel Swiller also shares his personal experiences with multiple life-threatening situations. He was comforted and found meaning in the strength of his attachments and the number of people who love him. He felt gratitude for the life he had lead. Finding meaning in the time remaining after one is told that one's life is in jeopardy is an important challenge for most patients. Many may need psychotherapy, medication, or spiritual guidance.

Finding meaning in one's final days is also a challenge for the therapist. We are especially indebted to the work of Victor Frankl's *Man's Search for Meaning* (1963 [1946]) and his writings on logotherapy. His works reflect his views on the role of meaning in permitting him to survive the death camp at Auschwitz. Survival in extreme circumstances depends on one's ability to find meaning in suffering. He outlines three categories of meaning: creative, on what one accomplishes or gives to the world; experiential, or what one takes from the world, that is, love, beauty, experiences; and finally, attitudinal, where one stands on a fate one cannot change, suffering (Frankl, 1963 [1946]). Facilitating a dying patient's attempts at meaning are an important way of avoiding demoralization and meaningless during suffering. They provide a means of transcending the suffering. William Breitbart and Karen Heller have instituted and studied the impact of meaning-centered group psychotherapy, which they discovered based on Frankl's logotherapy (Breitbart & Heller, 2003).

Similarly, a potent antidote to those who struggle with meaningless after confronting the transiency and finiteness of their existence is "rippling" (Yalom, 2008). Rippling results from the fact that each of us, without conscious intent or knowledge, exercises concentric circles of influence that may affect others for years, even for generations. A review of the journey of life has always been an important part of the content of many of my [Straker's] psychotherapeutic experiences with dying patients. It is very important for them to tell their life story, review the impact of their accomplishments and connections, and see the rippling.

Some have managed to find their own way, and they are great teachers. An example is from the biography of Steve Jobs. Walther Isaacson quotes Steve Jobs:

> Remembering that I will be dead soon is the most important tool I've encountered to help me make the big choices in my life. Because almost everything—all external expectations all pride, all fear of embarrassment or failure—these things just fall away in the face of death leaving only what is truly important. Remembering you're going to die is the best way to avoid the trap of thinking you have something to lose. You are already naked. There is no reason not to follow your heart. (Issacson, 2011)

Eugene O'Kelly offers a similar message in *Chasing Daylight: How My Forthcoming Death Transformed My Life* (2008). It is a book that can bring solace to those facing death. O'Kelly begins his book by noting the two questions he posed to himself after he was told he had three months to live: Why must the end of life be the worst part of life? And secondly, can it be made to be a constructive experience or even the best part? He felt that his experiences in the last few weeks were so meaningful that he had a strong need to share his planned experience in his book. This need to teach or speak of one's final journey is a frequent enough experience in my work that I think it is a part of the process that one goes through. It is a desire to share a life's experience, connect, and be remembered and validated before one is forever gone.

O'Kelly, in particular, felt the importance of taking control of the planning of how to live the last weeks—"to be the master of my own farewell." He made the decision, after careful consideration, to stop chemotherapy because it might prolong his life three months but deprive him of any quality. He resolved to live in the present, not in the future or the past, and try to "unwind relationships" by saying his goodbyes to all who had touched his life. He did this either by e-mail, phone, or in person. He was methodical, beginning with people who were more peripheral in his life and working toward his intimates for his final days. These meetings allowed him to remind himself of how many people he had touched and to honor the bond that connected them. He thanked them for their friendship and for sharing their talents and goodness. This experience helped him feel less alone and to realize that his life had touched many others.

AN EXTRAORDINARY EVENT

DANIEL BIRGER, MD

Like the Ancient Mariner, I feel a compulsion to write about the life-changing experience I went through during the last week of June and the first part of July 2011. My article will be composed of two different tracks. One will be the description of the events pertaining to my life-threatening illness, and the other will be my psychological reaction to it. In my discussion I will reflect on my understanding of the meaning of these events.

During the earlier part of June I felt more fatigued than usual but I continued my work and daily activities until I felt that I was developing flu. I had a few chills and unusual weakness and lost all my chess games to inferior players. I went to see my physician at his hospital office. He took a blood test. The next day, after seeing four patients in the morning, I received a phone call from him. "You have low white blood cells," he said. "Oh great," I replied, "it is only a viral flu." "No," he said, "it is *very* low. Come to the hospital now."

When I arrived, he ushered me directly to the hematology-oncology clinic and had the chief of the department look at my blood smear on the spot. The chief looked at me strangely and proclaimed, "You have no white blood cells." After examining a sample of my bone marrow under the microscope the chief said "Your bone marrow is empty, no cells. You stay here." I began to have a sense of concern and called my afternoon patients to cancel their sessions. Within an hour I was in the emergency room (ER), and my wife was there with me. There was no room in the hospital to which I could be admitted, so I had to stay in the emergency room. Being aware that I had no immunity, I got panicky, yelled at a nurse, and got put in a separate room in the ER. I remained there for twenty-four hours, getting sicker by the hour.

The next afternoon I was transferred to a room on the bone marrow transplant floor. I was in a state of disbelief: was I really that sick? The answer came fast and clearly in the form of intense chills. It is hard to describe the freezing sensation emanating from the core of my chest that threw me into violent shivering of every part of my body, accompanied by unbelievable misery. No amount of blankets helped the painful freezing sensation tormenting me. The episodes of chills were interspersed with episodes of high fever, which I recall less clearly. By that time, the doctors were swarming around me—infectious disease specialists, hemato-oncologists, internists, and transplant specialists. All seemed to be highly competent, first-rate doctors. I was punctured again for another bone marrow sample because they couldn't believe their eyes about the empty desolation of the first sample, but the second bone marrow produced the same results—emptiness.

Even though the days and nights seemed to be melded together, my conscious alertness remained intact. I didn't sleep much, and my mind talked to me with clarity about where I was, my predicament, and my condition. The chills kept coming, and I began to anticipate them with utter dread. Blood was drawn every few hours and cultures were sent. No specific cause of infection was found, but by that time I was under a wall-to-wall carpet of antibacterial, anti-fungal, and antiviral antibiotics. Steroids were pouring into the IV in whopping doses. The platelets were down from a normal 300,000 to only 7,000, and the white blood cell count was 200 instead of 6,000 to 10,000. The diagnosis was clear: aplastic anemia. During my medical school days, this was a swift death sentence.

It was a gradual process. But within four or five days in the hospital, it seemed as if my mind was expanding to absorb with more acuteness and relate with more intensity any communication with another person. My own thoughts assumed crystal clarity. My understanding was immediate; my conclusions seemed solid and indisputable. The expansion of the sense of consciousness and the bright luminosity with which my thoughts were endowed gave rise to a different sense of reality that was richer, more intense and, I dare say, more loving than I have ever felt before. My wife was beside my bed at every possible moment. My younger daughter was flying in from some distance. My other daughter and her husband came to see me at every opportunity they could find. My son kept calling with anxious questions about my condition. Between all of them I felt surrounded by love and I was comforted by their presence.

Clinically, the white blood cells were not moving, the platelets stagnant despite transfusions, and the chills persisted. The crew of physicians taking care of me was hardworking and dedicated, but despite all their efforts my clinical condition did not change much. The underlying process was autoimmune activity, triggered possibly by an allergy to an antibiotic or another unknown substance with which I had come into contact. My thymocytes, the cells that attack a foreign substance entering the body, were attacking and demolishing my own bone marrow. A decision was reached to treat me with ATG (antithymocyte globulin) to stem the autoimmune reaction. The ATG that was delivered intravenously was derived from horse serum. This brought about the most horrendous moment in the story of my illness: within a half hour I developed a galloping anaphylactic reaction, which brought me the closest I ever came to the grave. Gripped by monstrous chills, unable to breathe, I was shivering desperately. My oxygen saturation dropped to 30 percent. The group of doctors around me looked so worried that I felt the need to comfort them. "I am inhaling fine, "I said. "The only trouble is with the exhaling." They pulled me back from the hereafter by giving me oxygen, an epinephrine injection, and IV steroids. My hyper-acute mind reached the conclusion that I was going to die. I told my wife that when the time to go to the hospice came, she should take me to one that was close by so that she wouldn't have to travel far to see me.

About an hour and a half later, the anaphylaxis was gone, but my sprinting mind had been pushed into hyper drive. The acute clarity turned into a floodgate of blinding light, crystallizing into an awareness of a different quality and nature than I had ever had in my life. It is difficult to define its content, but its main quality was a sense of finality and an unshakable knowledge that I had reached the end of my life. Incongruously, that sense of conviction was not accompanied by an unpleasant effect. I did not experience terror, fear, or sadness. If anything, I can compare the effect to a feeling of welcoming rest after a long, arduous, productive, and gratifying day. My thoughts were that I had had a wonderful seventy-five years of life in which I had experienced a myriad of events and emotions, as well as collected knowledge, understanding, and fascinating interests. Most of all, I felt I was surrounded by the love of my family and the affection of my friends. I felt I was dying rich—rich with life experience, love, knowledge, pleasure, and having witnessed beauty.

I do not feel I had lost any sense of consciousness of events happening around me; I didn't become delusional or disoriented, but the quality with which I processed reality was intensified in an unfamiliar and wonderful way. I felt that the time left to me to be conscious should be devoted to my departure from my loved ones, family and friends. At this point, I want to stress again that as part of the treatment regimen I was receiving the equivalent of 380 milligrams of prednisone IV daily, which unquestionably affected the nature of my consciousness and no doubt created a hypomanic state.

The serenity with which I accepted my impending death did not last long. Like a floodgate opening wide came an onslaught of memories, the reviewing and evaluating of which compelled me to recall and relive moments of my life. At first, the flow was quite chaotic but then some orderly, chronological, organized pattern emerged and took control of the process. Some of the memories came in visual form and some with the quality of reminiscence, but all had a vivid emotional intensity attached to them, as if I was living the moment of their occurrence. No material with which I was unfamiliar in the past appeared in my consciousness: these were experiences that were never repressed but had faded into the fog that we leave behind as we move on in our lives. However, the vividness of the experience was something I had never felt before.

With the inner pulsating pressure of the memories came an irresistible compulsion to talk in pressured, non-stop speech, describing each memory to whoever would listen. I was weak and exhausted, but I could not stop breath-lessly describing my inner experience. I did not pay heed to the fact that my family members started getting a strange expression when I assaulted them relentlessly with my memories—the compulsion of the Ancient Mariner con-trolled me.

When the doctors started reducing the steroid level, I gained more control but the urge continued in a mitigated way. The clinical condition took a turn for the better after a successful treatment with ATG derived from rabbit serum, which was not rejected by my body. All signs of septicemia were gone, and the bone marrow began to show signs of life in response to the treatment. But that did not modify my conviction that I was in the process of dying.

A new attitude toward the people surrounding me became very apparent. I became hyper-interested in the staff. Nurses, nurses aides, cleaning staff— each became a unique individual of different background—most of them foreign-born—Filipinos, Koreans, Caribbeans, South Americans—I asked them about their lives, families, and their adaptation to life here. They eager-ly told me about their families, their gratifications and disappointments, and I felt a sense of connection that was unusually strong with people I was just getting to know.

I felt so safe in being taken care of by the staff that I found myself having hypnagogic hallucinations that there were staff members surrounding me and taking care of me. But when I opened my eyes, there was no one there.

The relationship with the medical staff was experienced with a special glow. My personal physician, who is also my friend, was involved with my case throughout its course, coming to visit daily, communicating needs and information to other specialists, and trying to fulfill any request or answer any questions I had. I could barely contain my sense of gratitude. The hema-to-oncologist who conducted the treatment also showed superb dedication and confidence. The infectious disease expert who relieved me of my septi-cemia with his concoction of antibiotics bounded into my room daily with a cheerful smile under his mustache and always an encouraging word.

The family devotion I have mentioned was continuous. My visiting younger daughter sat beside me. My wife was efficient, effective, and watch-ful for all my needs. My older daughter and her hard-working husband were beside me every evening. My granddaughters, worried by my appearance and intimidated by the atmosphere by the hospital, nonetheless delivered me a lot of affection. All were a source of comfort for me. My friends and family from home kept calling, anxious and offering all good wishes for me.

Friends' visits and phone calls met me in a state of open receptivity and uninhibited ability to express my gratitude for their friendship. Their support provided a powerful sense, enhanced by steroids, of being liked, loved, and respected.

My clinical condition continued to improve, and with that, the compulsion to tell my story became somewhat mitigated. The combination of effective medications nudged my bone marrow to show signs of life as white blood cells reappeared in gradually growing numbers. My conviction about my impending death began showing cracks of doubt, which turned into cautious hope as my improvement continued by leaps and bounds. The blood counts improved daily and there began to be vague talk of sending me home.

I began to believe that I had gotten a great gift—a bonus of time in which to live more of my life. And my cup of gratitude started running over. The hypomania due to steroids persisted in two particular ways: first, my debilitating insomnia; and then hyper excitation and an indiscriminate intensity of response to any call of greeting and well wishing from friends or acquaintances, as if I wanted to infect them with my enthusiasm about the miracle of my regaining my life. I realized the inappropriateness of my responses but I couldn't help it most of the time.

After three weeks in the hospital I was discharged back home. There I found a solution to the pressure to tell my story. I pounced on a pad of paper and poured out my memories like an avalanche. Writing five or six hours a night made me feel very productive. Eventually, after putting on paper a lot of my life story in a cathartic way, I felt empty and exhausted but exhilarated and free of the pressure. Blessed be the steroid insomnia!

Reflections on My Confrontation with Death

I realize that I have told two stories. One is the story of my illness; the other, my psychological reactions to it.

It is clear to me that the urgent compulsive onslaught of my life stories had multiple functions for me. On the most apparent level it was what I consciously considered it to be—an evaluation of my path in life, coming to the conclusion that I have lived a full life. I knew defeat and failure, and I knew resilience and success. I knew love, and I knew hate. I knew attachment, and I knew the pain of separation and loss. On the whole, looking at the trajectory of my life, I see that I have walked a long way from the point where I started to the point that I anticipated to be the end of my road. I accumulated knowledge, experience, and, hopefully, wisdom. I managed to curb and sublimate my aggression, and continued to evolve, to absorb new ideas, and to enjoy art and literature. I have traveled a lot and seen the beauty of this world. I continued to mature without losing the playful child in me.

I also needed such a positive evaluation in order to reassure myself that my life had been a worthwhile experience, that death could not deprive me of a life already fully and productively lived. This was a comforting conclusion, comforting enough to enable me to feel a sense of equanimity in the face of what I thought was the end of my being. I have no doubt that the hypomanic state induced by the vast quantities of steroids pouring into my veins helped a great deal in preventing feelings of terror and desperation I might have felt facing my death. However, the content of my mind was my own psychological working system The steroids certainly affected my mood, the quality of my consciousness, my exaggerated loving feelings toward my surroundings, and the compulsivity of my speech. But this did not distort my cognitive accuracy or the reality of my memories. Even today, free of steroid treatment for months, I stand by my memories and my conclusion about life.

Finally, exploring the experience with the tools of psychodynamic inquiry gives more depth and dimensionality to my understanding of the functions that reviewing my life served for me. As I go over the events described in my memories, I realize that many of those events carried a feeling of danger for me of extreme challenges, the threat of thwarting me, defeating me, preventing my progress. Such memories might have been motivated by my desire to overcome the present menace as well, as though to say to myself, "I overcame those past challenges, I can overcome this one too." Even though on the surface I felt I was accepting death with equanimity, a part of me was fighting unconsciously against the verdict by eliciting the hope that I would prevail in this battle too.

Also, regarding the quality of clinging in my communications, I view it as a good example of the difficulty to tease apart the biological effect of the steroids from the psychological struggle represented in my Ancient Mariner syndrome. As well as being a hypomanic behavior caused by the steroids, it also showed a clinging to life through communication with others. Any visitor or person who called on the phone became the target of my incessant and urgent need to talk. So, again, despite a conscious belief that I was resigned to parting from this world, I believe that there was a part of me trying to cling to life by holding on to other people, grasping for their attention like a drowning man grasps at any lifeline.

The flood of memories had at least two functions. Primarily, it was for me to reassure myself that I had had a full, successful life and that death was not cheating me of anything. But it also served another purpose, in that the compulsion to tell it to others bound me to life through possessing their attention, a sort of Scheherazade defense mechanism.

My tale may reflect a subjective unique experience of coping with a powerful threat of imminent death over a period of weeks. Others may employ different defense mechanisms, but most have not returned to tell about their experience. I hope my returning to tell the tale may add some insight into the complex question of how humans attempt to cope with the inevitability of ceasing to be.

Addendum

I am writing this chapter exactly a year after the date of my hospitalization. It was a wonderful year. I have a sense that every new day is a gift. I returned to work with my patients, hopefully wiser than before, but I also dedicate more time to pleasurable activities. I resigned from some voluntary commitments I had before the illness and cherish more time spent with my loved ones. The return of my physical well-being enabled me to experience uplifting events such as going to ski in the West, gliding on the white slopes under the brilliant blue sky, blessing every moment for the miracle of life.

I have read more books, seen more plays, and enjoyed playing more games, acknowledging the bliss of being in this world. Just recently I returned from a bicycle trip in Holland. Riding along canals, beside huge green fields with spotted cows, passing windmills jutting up to the bright blue sky, I drank with joy every drop of the excitement of being alive. I wonder if I would have appreciated it with such intensity if I had not had the experience of coming face-to-face with death, close enough to look into the darkness of its hollow eye sockets, and yet return to the sunshine of life.

ON ILLNESS AND DEATH

HILLEL SWILLER, MD

It was the best of times, it was the worst of times . . . it was the season of Light, it was the season of Darkness, it was the spring of hope, it was the winter of despair . . .

—Charles Dickens, *A Tale of Two Cities*

It began not at the moment I discovered my first cancer, a bulge in my neck, but a day later when the young ears, nose, and throat (ENT) specialist who confirmed the diagnosis said, in an attempt to comfort me, "Life sucks." My spontaneous reply was, "I've had a good life."

So it began: a journey of illness and an exploration of meaning and value in my sixty-sixth year. Over the past few years, I have endured radiation therapy resulting in four months of being unable to swallow (requiring feeding through a peg tube), chemotherapy (causing a major hearing loss), a modified radical neck dissection, an aortic valve transplant, colon cancer (leading to a partial resection of my colon), a fungal septicemia (for which I received inadequate treatment at a local hospital and would have been sent home with a growth on my valve ripe for an embolus had my wife not insisted on my transfer to my own medical center), a second aortic valve replacement, a cardiac arrest, a prostatectomy (the most painful surgery of all), and a stroke (taking much of the vision in my right eye). I may have left something out, but you get the picture.

My friends and colleagues tell me they are struck by my resilience, which is why I have been asked to write this chapter. How have I done this? The answer is rather simple to express, although perhaps not always so simple to implement.

"I've had a good life," I said on that second day, and so I have. I think about that often. I try to practice gratitude. I am, and if you are reading this, you probably are as well, a citizen of the United States. This is a totally unearned piece of good fortune. Because of this I have had the unfettered opportunity to live, as so few others have had, in security, abundance, and the ability to go as far as my talents and energy would take me. I have a more personal list as well. Forty-six years ago, I married out of blind unthinking lust and it has turned out to be the smartest decision I have ever made. I have wonderful children and grandchildren. My extended family is warm and nurturing. I have many wonderful friends. (Two simple ideas have aided in this. One, to have a friend, be a friend. Two, don't keep score. I never hesitate to be the one to make the call.) I have a fascinating and fulfilling professional life. There's more, but I think you get the picture. I am a most lucky fellow.

My journey sent me back not just to my personal psychology but to philosophy as well. First, I revisited Ernest Becker's classic *The Denial of Death*. Psychiatrists have relatively neglected this powerful book, but some of our colleagues in social psychology have done wonderful work building on it. Irvin Yalom's writings have been of great interest and help to me since the time I was a psychiatric resident. His recent volume, *Staring at the Sun*, is an explicit exploration of the experience of confronting death. Yalom led me back to many of the profound thinkers throughout history. I can't begin to summarize the accumulated wisdom I have mined as a result. (Another thing for which I am grateful is having had several wonderful teachers and mentors.) A few of the ideas that have benefited me are that death is inevitable and unknowable and to be accepted as such. We did not exist before birth and we won't exist after death. With death comes an end to all suffering. Loss is inherent in life; we lose those we love until they lose us; we lose function and vigor. What do you do? You do what you can. We live in a random universe without external purpose or meaning. It is the task for each of us to create the meaning that will sustain us. We do this by imposing our will upon our circumstances. We cannot control much of what reality presents to us, but we can choose how we respond. Does this mean that I believe in free will? My answer is far from original: of course I believe in free will; what choice do I have? I'm back where I started: I have created meaning for myself through family, friends, and work. That sustains me. I try to live in the moment and extract from each moment all that I can.

I shouldn't end without addressing the issue of depression. If I seem to have suggested that through all this I have had no depression, I have misled you. Depression, not sadness, from which it usually can be differentiated, has come and gone over the years. I experience it as a wave of physical sensation. Thinking in depression is secondary, superficial, and a form of rationalization. We can be sad about something, but depression lives beneath thought. I accept it as such and as I do the inevitability of death. The physical wave will, in time, recede; in time, my life will end. That's just the way it is.

My journey over these last few years has provided me with many kinds of pain, but it has also enabled me to learn how to minimize suffering and to be content.

REFERENCES

Breitbart, W., & Heller K. S. (2003). Reframing hope: Meaning-centered care for patients near the end of life. *Journal of Palliative Medicine, 6*(6).

Frankl, V. (1963 [1946]). *Man's search for meaning*. Boston: Beacon Press.

———. (1972). The feeling of meaninglessness: A challenge to psychotherapy. *American Journal of Psychoanalysis, 32*, 82–85.

———. (1969). The will to meaning. *New York World*.

Heidegger, M. (2008 [1927]). *Being and time: Death transformed my life*. New York: Harper & Row.

Hutchinson, T. A., Mount, B. M., & Kearney, M. (2011). The healing journey. In T. A. Hutchinson (Ed.), *Whole person care: A new paradigm for the 21st century*. Quebec: Springer.

Isaacson, W. (2011). *Steve Jobs*. New York: Simon & Schuster.

Kierkegaard, S. (1957). *The concept of dread*. Princeton: Princeton University Press.

O'Kelly, E. (2008). *Chasing daylight: How my forthcoming death transformed my life*. New York: McGraw Hill.

Tolstoy, L. (1931). *War and peace*. New York: Modern Library.

———. (1960). *The death of Ivan Ilych and other stories*. New York: Signet Classics.

Yalom, I. (2008). *Staring at the sun: Overcoming the fear of death*. San Francisco: Wiley.

II

Psychoanalytic Section

Chapter Four

The Denial of the Fear of Death by Psychoanalysts

Norman Straker, MD

Recent research on "death anxiety" and the current clinical practice in the treatment of patients facing death recommends an update in the psychoanalytic literature. The following chapter, "Finding Meaning in Death: Terror Management among the Terminally Ill," reviews the empirical research on death anxiety. The case reports by analysts that follow will illustrate current psychoanalytic practice for analysts treating cancer patients who are facing death.

My own training analysis is the example par excellence of how facing death was formerly avoided in clinical work and possibly still is today by those analysts who have limited exposure to dying patients and the current expanded psychoanalytic literature. Memories of my experience only came to mind while I was writing the first draft of this book.

During my early thirties, during my training analysis, I had been hospitalized for respiratory failure from viral pneumonia. My analyst had declined to be in contact with me during either my hospitalization or recuperation. He explained to my wife on the telephone, "I do not want to introduce the human element into the analysis." On my return to the analysis, I recall a session in which I was reviewing my experience in the hospital. I described how I had attributed psychological meaning to my breathlessness and wheezing. Earlier in my career, I had conducted research on the relationship between repressed aggression in children and bronchial asthma. While my analyst said nothing at the time about my hospital experience, it is now clear to me, in retrospect, that I was trying to deny my helplessness and my fears of suffocating to death. I was attributing psychological meaning to my symptoms and trying to improve my breathing by psychoanalyzing myself. These experiences were of no particular interest to my psychoanalyst. He asked no questions and made no comment. This is not an indictment of him, but customary practice at that time, which I expect and hope is less common today.

What might be the reason that Freudian psychoanalysts have written so little about the importance of the fear of death? Perhaps it has something to do with the old cliché that doctors who are afraid of blood and death become psychiatrists and psychoanalysts. More likely, it is a legacy of Freudian theory. This avoidance of facing death or denial of the fear of death has roots in Sigmund Freud's writing. Freud gave little importance to the fear of death.

Despite the fact that Freud's early cases had illness or death as a very integral part of their history, he gave no theoretical importance to those facts; Fraulein Elizabeth became ill after her father and sister died, Anna O. developed her illness while tending to her father who was terminally ill, and finally, Frau Emmy von N became ill after her husband's death (Breuer & Freud, 1895). Irvin Yalom suggests that it took a supreme effort of inattention for Freud to have omitted death as a precipitating factor in these early cases of hysteria (Yalom, 1980).

> It is indeed impossible to imagine our own death; and whenever we attempt to do so we can perceive that we are in fact still present as spectators. Hence the psychoanalytic school could venture on the assertion that at bottom no one believes in his own death or to put the same thing in another way, that in the unconscious everyone is convinced of his own immortality. . . . It is questionable whether there is any such thing as a normal fear of death; actually the idea of death is subjectively inconceivable and therefore probably every fear of death covers other unconscious ideas. (Freud, 1915)

In *Symptoms, Inhibitions, and Anxiety*, Freud dismissed the fear of death as a superficial fear; a derivative of the genetic fears of childhood. He believed that since we have no direct experience with death, we couldn't fear it.

> But the unconscious seems to contain nothing that could give any content to our concept of the annihilation of life. Castration can be pictured on the daily experience of the feces being separated from the body. . . . But nothing resembling death can ever have been experienced. . . . I am therefore inclined to adhere to the view that the fear of death should be regarded as analogous to the fear of castration and that the situation to which the ego is reacting is one of being abandoned by the protecting super ego . . . (Freud, 1926)

Yalom believes that Freud was a prisoner of his deterministic system; death being a future event that had never been experienced cannot exist in the unconscious and therefore cannot influence behavior (Yalom, 1980). Freud could speak of death off the record, however, as in *Our Attitude toward Death*, in which he wrote of man's attempt to vanquish death through immortality myths (Freud, 1915). In a brief essay, "On Transience" (1916), Freud conveys a perspective on mortality that was not integrated into his theoretical systems. In the article, he writes about the "foretaste of mourning" that is experienced in considering the transience of cherished things. Irwin Hoffman (1979) considers this to be a bridge to existentially oriented views that will follow in existentialism.

Freud's theoretical positions on this issue have had the unfortunate result of having psychoanalysts believe that the fear of death is derived only from the genetic fears of childhood. This idea perpetuates the view that working through childhood conflicts allows for all anxiety to be subject to extinction. Death anxiety, which is unfixable and not analyzable, is, in fact, problematic. As we will see later, the analyst who works with dying patients and tries to analyze the patient's fear of death using Freudian views will not extinguish death anxiety and, in fact, will feel personally anxious and impotent.

A contrasting view is held by Yalom (1980) who says, "The fear of death plays a major role in our experience; . . . it rumbles continuously under the surface; it is a dark, unsettling presence at the rim of consciousness." While we are certainly aware of the reality of death as it may impact others, we are able to deny its risks to ourselves using two defensive fantasies. One is our sense of specialness that makes us inviolable, allowing us to believe we are the exception. To the extent that one achieves power, achieves wealth, leaves important work behind, or is a doctor, one's anxiety is assuaged. The other is our belief in the ultimate rescuer, God, or the omnipotence of our doctor. "It is not as if one really denies that death exists . . . it just is not in the cards for me because I am special because . . . or I am protected by . . . God or my most expert doctor" (Yalom, 1980).

Patients who are in terror or panic after they have been told they have cancer or that their cancer is incurable often lose their capacity to deny and often seek out a psychoanalyst for treatment. Death anxiety cannot be analyzed away as a derivative of childhood conflict; it must be faced head-on. This challenge can make the inexperienced analysts, therapists, or psychiatrists very uncomfortable. The primary motivation for analysts attending my discussion group of thirty years, "Psychoanalysis and Psychodynamic Psychotherapy of Cancer Patients" at the American Psychoanalytic Meetings, is countertransference reactions to facing death. Anxiousness about the analyst's own death, identification with a dying patient, especially if he or she is close in age, or feelings of impotence are the most common challenges. These feelings create concerns about how to respond to the patient's distress—how to talk about death, if and how the analyst should alter his technique, should they see family members, interface with the medical staff, attend funerals after the patient dies, and so forth. The individual case reports in this book were all presented at this discussion group. They help to provide an updated approach for psychoanalysts who will treat patients facing death. Three case reports primarily focus on countertransference issues.

At one of these meetings, a young female analyst, the mother of two young children, presented a woman about her age who was dying of metastatic breast cancer. The analyst (Alison C. Phillips) found the sessions overwhelmingly painful emotionally as her patient began to confront her death and the impending loss of her two young daughters. These girls were exactly the same age as the analyst's two girls. The analyst was not only identifying with the patient and her girls, but she was also suffering from unconscious survivor guilt. The group was helpful in pointing out the difficult issues for the analyst and supporting her work (see chapter 10).

At another meeting, an analytic candidate with breast cancer (Patricia Plopa) reported that during the height of her own fear of dying, her training analyst initially took the position that she (the training analyst) was sure her patient would survive. At that time, the analytic candidate experienced this reassurance as very supportive. However, this avoidance of anxiety for both of them delayed an exploration of the patient's fear of death until a later time. Further reading of Dr. Plopa's chapter reveals that indeed there were opportunities for her to face her fear of death (see chapter 12).

To some degree, we analysts, like everyone else, are troubled by our impotence when it comes to confronting our patients' death anxiety. Some analysts, even I, colluded with patients and retreated from directly talking about death, rationalizing that, as Freud had suggested, patients believe in their own immortality. However, I now realize that when patients are facing death directly, we need to be with them and help them. We need to choose the appropriate moment when death anxiety is preconscious or conscious rather than when it is highly defended. I will refer to what I term a commonsense approach to denial in chapter 7. I have learned that an acceptance of my own mortality and a calm demeanor can create a holding environment that allows for an exploration of all the issues that confront dying patients. The view that death anxiety is an existential anxiety, with contributions from early childhood derivatives, leads to a more effective approach in helping patients facing death and will be elaborated by the contributing authors of this book.

REFERENCES

Breuer, J., & Freud, S. (1895). *Studies on hysteria, 2.* London: The Hogarth Press, 135–183.
Freud, S. (1915). *Thoughts for our times, 14.* London: The Hogarth Press, 299.
———. (1916). *On transience, 14.* London: The Hogarth Press, 303.
———. (1926). *Symptoms, inhibitions, and anxiety, 20.* London: The Hogarth Press, 1.
Hoffman, I. (1979). Death, anxiety, and the adaptation to mortality in psychoanalytic theory. *Annual of Psychoanalysis, 7,* 233–267.
Solomon, S., Greenberg, J., & Pyszczynski, T. (1998). Tales from the crypt: On the role of death in life. *Zygon, 33*(1), 9–43.
Yalom, I. D. (1980). *Existential psychotherapy.* New York: Basic Books.

Chapter Five

Finding Meaning in Death

Terror Management among the Terminally Ill

Molly Maxfield, Tom Pyszczynski, and
Sheldon Solomon

For most people, "a good death" would come in one's sleep without pain, conscious awareness, or fear, after a long and satisfying life filled with meaning, value, and love. Unfortunately, death comes far too soon for many. For those diagnosed with terminal illness, death often follows arduous and painful medical treatments, isolated from the routines of normal living within the confines of a hospital. Terminal diagnoses force people to confront the reality of their own personal mortality not as an abstract problem for the distant future but as a pressing immediate concern. Although everyone knows they will someday die, the emotional impact of this awareness is typically blunted by a host of psychological defenses that defuse the potential for terror that this knowledge entails. Indeed, terror management theory, or TMT (Greenberg, Pyszczynski, & Solomon, 1986; Solomon, Greenberg, & Pyszczynski, 1991), posits that awareness of the inevitability of death has a profound influence on much of what people think, feel, and do, and is the primary impetus for the human pursuit of meaning, value, and love. In this chapter, we use TMT as a framework to consider how people cope with terminal illness, with a focus on factors that foster more and less adaptive coping with the many challenges resulting from such diagnoses.

From this perspective, knowledge of the inevitability of death is a major existential problem that has a profound influence on all people at all stages of life. As William James (1890) put it, death is the "worm at the core," a deep underlying fear that drives people even when they are not particularly aware of it as a problem. TMT research has shown that when people are reminded of death, they cling more tenaciously to their cultural worldviews, work harder to attain and maintain self-esteem, and show increased desire for close intimate connections with other people. Interestingly, this increased need for security emerges not while people are consciously contemplating their mortality, but when such thoughts are on the fringes of consciousness, easily called to mind but not what they are actively thinking about. And these effects are consistently found in people who are young and in good health with every reason to expect many years of life ahead of them, for whom death is typically thought of as an abstract problem for the distant future. But what about people for whom death is a more immediate and pressing concern?

We have much more to learn about how terror management processes operate among people who are close to death. But we have recently begun investigating this question in two lines of research: one focused on people who have had traumatic life experiences in which imminent death was a very real possibility, and the other focused on older adults in their final decades of life. Traumatic life events such as war, terrorism, interpersonal violence, earthquakes, and other various natural and manmade disasters often pose sudden and violent threats to a person's continued survival. Although most people adapt reasonably well to such traumatic experiences, others experience an array of devastating psychological disturbances collectively referred to as posttraumatic stress disorder (PTSD). Our research suggests that PTSD occurs when the traumatic event leads to a serious disruption or collapse of the normal anxiety-buffering functions of cultural worldviews, self-esteem, and close interpersonal attachments (Pyszczynski & Kesebir, 2011). The normal aging process, on the other hand, affords people a relatively gradual progression toward death, with decades to adapt to and prepare for the inevitable end of life. Indeed, important teachings within most religious traditions suggest that one of the primary goals of life is to prepare oneself for death by learning the "art of dying." We have recently begun exploring the processes through which older adults come to grips with their rapidly increasing proximity to death (e.g., Maxfield et al., 2007). This research suggests that some people go through a developmental transition in later life that enables them to approach death in a less fearful and rigidly defensive manner. These changes in coping strategies might be responsible for the relatively high levels of psychological well-being found in some but not all older adults (for a review, see Charles & Carstensen, 2010). Though focused on very different problems, these two lines of inquiry can be thought of as exemplifying the negative and positive ways in which more direct and personal confrontations with death can affect people's anxiety-buffering systems. Both of these lines of research also suggest, perhaps not surprisingly, that people differ widely in how they respond to situations that make death a very immediate and pressing problem.

Research and clinical observations similarly tell us that people vary mark-edly in how they cope with the knowledge of impending death that comes with terminal diagnoses. Although many people respond to terminal diagno-sis with overwhelming terror, depression, and despair, others cope reason-ably well, and some even show signs of growth and increased psychological well-being (e.g., Kübler-Ross, 1969). Unfortunately, to date we know of no studies that have used the TMT framework to explore what leads to more and less successful coping with terminal illness. Given what TMT research has revealed about how people cope with death when it is *not* an immediate pressing problem and *can* be construed as a problem for the distant future, along with the changes in these coping processes that that emerge after exposure to trauma and in the later years of life, it seems likely that TMT could shed useful insights into what leads to more and less favorable adapta-tion to terminal illness.

TERROR MANAGEMENT THEORY (TMT)

TMT was inspired by the work of cultural anthropologist Ernest Becker, who, in *The Denial of Death* (1973), explored the distinctively human prob-lem of awareness of the inevitability of death. When juxtaposed with the drive for survival ingrained within all species, this awareness creates the potential for paralyzing terror that would seriously undermine other adaptive behavior and make consciousness unbearably aversive. Our ancestors adapted to this potential for terror by imbuing their emerging conceptions of reality with cosmic significance. These humanly created cultural worldviews to enable people to manage their fear of death by construing themselves as valuable contributors to a meaningful and enduring universe. By immersing themselves in the ongoing cultural drama, people are able to avert the anxiety that would result from more direct consideration of the inevitability of death.

As part of their death-denying cultural worldviews, humankind invented meaningful narratives for the origins of the universe, the purpose of life, and the means by which to gain both literal and symbolic immortality. Literal immortality refers to the belief that life continues in some form after physical death, in heaven or other supernatural realms, through reincarnation, or by means of some form of unification with the spirits of other departed beings. Symbolic immortality refers to the sense that one is part of something greater than oneself that will last forever; it is attained by making valued and endur-ing contributions to the cultural reality, for example, by creating works of art or science, building monuments, or amassing great fortunes. Cultural world-views also specify which behaviors are worthy of reward and punishment, both in this life and after death. Thus, people are protected from the existen-tial terror that awareness of death would otherwise produce by maintaining faith in their cultural worldviews and attaining self-esteem by living up to the standards of value that their worldviews provide. Consequently, people are powerfully motivated to maintain the meaning that their worldviews provide and the self-esteem that they get when they live up to the standards and values of worldviews. For a more thorough discussion of TMT and the role that death plays in diverse aspects of life, see Solomon, Greenberg, and Pyszczynski (1998).

To date, well over five hundred studies conducted in diverse cultures and locations have supported hypotheses derived from TMT. The mortality salience hypothesis suggests that to the extent one's cultural worldview and self-esteem are important buffers against existential anxiety, then these buffers will become even more valued and important when people are reminded of their mortality. In the first test of the mortality salience hypothesis (Rosenblatt, Greenberg, Solomon, Pyszczynski, & Lyon, 1989), municipal court judges were asked questions about mortality or a control topic and were then given a sample court case involving a woman arrested for prostitution for which they were instructed to assign bail. Because of their extensive training in the legal and justice systems, it can be assumed that following the law was an essential part of the judges' cultural worldviews. In support of the mortality salience hypothesis, judges reminded of mortality recommended significantly harsher bond ($455) compared to the judges in the control condition ($50), suggesting that thoughts of death lead to increased defense and affirmation of the cultural worldview. Other studies have shown that mortality salience increases positive evaluations of those who uphold or share one's worldview and negative evaluations of those who challenge one's worldview or hold alternative worldviews (Greenberg et al., 1990), increases self-esteem striving and defensive denial of failures (Mikulincer & Florian, 2002), and increases commitment to close relationships (e.g., Mikulincer, Florian, & Hirschberger, 2003).

Interestingly, self-reported fear of death is unrelated to responses to these reminders of mortality. In most mortality salience studies, participants report that they are not afraid of death; most are unaware that death had anything to do with their behavior in the study. In fact, one study revealed that lower self-reported fear of death predicted greater defensiveness following a reminder of death (Greenberg et al., 1995), suggesting that maintaining the integrity of their anxiety-buffering worldviews, self-esteem, and attachments helps people deny the fact that the problem of their mortality bothers them. Indeed, research has shown that people with anxiety disorders, who presumably have poorly functioning anxiety buffers, respond to reminders of death by showing greater phobic, compulsive, and avoidance reactions to other things that frighten them, such as spiders, contamination, or social interaction (Strachan et al., 2007). Research has also shown that giving people a placebo that is believed to block their ability to experience anxiety eliminates the effect of death reminders on subsequent defensive responses (Greenberg et al., 2003). Taken together, these studies suggest that it is the potential for anxiety rather than consciously experienced distress that motivates mainte- nance of the anxiety-buffering system.

Research has also shown that boosting self-esteem or faith in one's worldview reduces self-reports of anxiety, physiological arousal, and defen- sive distortions that deny one's vulnerability to death (e.g., Greenberg et al., 1993). Similarly, threats to self-esteem or one's worldview increase the ac- cessibility of death-related but not other aversive thoughts (for a review, see Hayes, Schimel, Arndt, & Faucher, 2010). For example, Canadian students who read an essay criticizing Canada and fundamentalist Christian students who read an essay supporting evolution were more likely to complete word stems in a death-related way; for example, the word stem COFF_ _ was more likely to be completed as COFFIN than COFFEE (Schimel, Hayes, Williams, & Jahrig, 2007). For recent reviews of the TMT literature, see Greenberg, Solomon, and Arndt (2008).

People use very different tactics to cope with the problem of death, de- pending on whether it is in current focal attention or not (Pyszczynski, Greenberg, & Solomon, 1999). When people are consciously aware of the problem of death, they use proximal defenses, which attack the threat in a more or less logical and rational manner. For example, immediately follow- ing reminders of death, while such thoughts are still in conscious attention, young adults report increased intention to engage in health-promoting behav- iors such as more frequent exercise (Arndt, Schimel, & Goldenberg, 2003) and sunscreen use (Routledge, Arndt, & Goldenberg, 2004). Sometimes peo- ple simply suppress death-related thoughts when they arise, pushing them out of consciousness by seeking distractions or self-medicating with alcohol or other substances (e.g., Arndt, Greenberg, Solomon, Pyszczynski, & Simon, 1997). Distal defenses, on the other hand, do not appear to be related to the problem of mortality in any logical or semantic sense. Recommending a harsher punishment for a prostitute, for example, does not actually solve the problem of death; rather, it affirms and strengthens faith in one's anxiety- buffering cultural worldview. Distal defenses involving the pursuit of mean- ing and self-esteem occur when thoughts of death are accessible but not in focal attention, or when death reminders are presented subtly (e.g., Arndt, Greenberg, Pyszczynski, & Solomon, 1997). Research has shown that distal defenses involving worldview, self-esteem, and attachment reduce both the accessibility of death-related thoughts and the need to engage in other forms of defense against the problem of death.

The TMT literature documents the pervasive impact that the problem of death has in diverse aspects of everyday life for people who are not in particular danger of dying anytime soon. As noted above, these processes change when people confront more immediate threats to their mortality, as in the case of traumatic life events and normal aging. We now turn to recent research on these issues.

COPING WITH DEATH AFTER TRAUMATIC LIFE EVENTS

Traumatic events, especially those involving the possible death of oneself or one's loved ones, challenge the belief that the world is safe and benevolent (Janoff-Bulman, 1992). If one's worldview and personal value are unable to provide protection against terrible events, then one's anxiety-buffering mechanisms may be seriously disrupted or entirely collapse, thus leaving one unprotected from anxiety (Pyszczynski & Kesebir, 2011). Anxiety-buffer disruption theory, or ABDT (Abdollahi, Pyszczynski, Maxfield, & Luszczynska, 2011; Pyszczynski & Kesebir, 2011), is an extension of TMT to the processes involved in coping with trauma. ABDT posits that traumatic experiences lead to PTSD when they produce a major disruption or collapse of the anxiety-buffering functioning of a person's worldview, self-esteem, and close attachments.

PTSD is a severely debilitating anxiety disorder that results from experiencing, witnessing, or confronting events that involve actual or threatened death or serious injury (American Psychiatric Association [DSM-IV-TR], 2000). Violent personal assaults, natural or human-caused disasters, accidents, and military combat are among the most commonly encountered triggers of the disorder; serious medical problems, including the diagnosis and treatment of terminal illness are increasingly recognized as another common trigger of PTSD (for a review, see Tedstone & Tarrier, 2003). People suffering from PTSD report recurrent re-experiencing of the traumatic event in flashbacks, nightmares, and intrusive thoughts; avoidance of reminders of the traumatic event; generalized numbing of emotional responses; and heightened arousal, as evidenced by hyper-vigilance, sleep disturbances, and exaggerated startle responses. The overall picture of the PTSD-afflicted person is suggestive of a person struggling with recurrent bouts of overwhelming terror.

ABDT posits that the damage to the anxiety-buffering system, and thus the severity of posttraumatic symptoms, depends on both the severity of the trauma and the prior strength and robustness of the individual's anxiety-buffering system. Less severe or more distantly experienced traumas experienced by persons with hardy anxiety-buffering systems are likely to stress the system but lead to exaggerated attempts to maintain faith in one's worldview, self-esteem, and relationships. This seems to be how the vast majority of Americans responded to the 9/11 terrorist attacks—ingroup unity, anger toward those perceived as threatening to the culture, increased patriotism, attempts to help those directly affected, and desire for the comfort of loving relationships—but relatively rare occurrences of diagnosable PTSD, estimated at 7.5 percent for those living in Manhattan at the time of the attacks (Galea et al., 2002) and 5.8 percent for Americans in general (Silver, Holman, McIntosh, Poulin, & Gil-Rivas, 2002). However, severe traumas experienced by those with more fragile anxiety-buffering systems produce major disruptions or even collapse of the anxiety-buffering system, and therefore to clinically significant PTSD.

A growing body of evidence documents the role of disrupted anxiety-buffer functioning in PTSD (for a review, see Pyszczynski & Kesebir, 2011). Among survivors of a devastating earthquake in Iran, extent of peritraumatic dissociation (psychologically disengaging during the traumatic event) predicted disrupted anxiety-buffer responses to reminders of both mortality and the earthquake itself one month after the quake (Abdollahi et al., 2011). Whereas persons with low levels of dissociation showed the typical elevation of worldview defense and no increase in negative affect in response to mortality salience, those with high levels of dissociation did not engage in typical worldview defense and showed elevated negative affect following reminders of mortality or the earthquake. Two years after the event, atypical responses to mortality salience were found among those with clinically significant levels of PTSD, but typical worldview defenses were found among those with low levels of PTSD symptoms. As in previous research (e.g., Ozer, Best, Lipsey, & Weiss, 2003), peritraumatic dissociation assessed one month after the event was associated with higher levels of PTSD symptoms two years later. Importantly, this relationship between dissociation and symptom severity was mediated by disrupted anxiety-buffer functioning.

Similar results were found in a study conducted in Poland with survivors of domestic violence (Kesebir, Luszczynska, Pyszczynski, & Benight, 2011). Whereas people with low levels of either PTSD symptom severity or particular predictors of PTSD, specifically high peritraumatic dissociation or low coping self-efficacy (e.g., Benight & Bandura, 2004), showed the typical mortality salience effect of harsher judgments of moral transgressions, those with high levels of PTSD or either of these predictors of PTSD showed the atypical response of more lenience toward moral transgressions in response to mortality reminders. In another series of studies conducted following the Ivory Coast civil war (Chatard et al., 2012), researchers found that people with more severe PTSD symptoms displayed an absence of the usual suppression of death-related thoughts immediately following a reminder of death, whereas those with low levels of symptoms showed the suppression of such thoughts that has been found in many previous studies of non-traumatized persons. In a second study with this population, individuals with greater exposure to the war reported more severe PTSD symptoms when reminded of mortality whereas participants with low exposure to war responded to mortality salience with reduced reports of PTSD symptoms. Because exaggerating one's well-being is a common defensive response to existential threat, this is further evidence that PTSD is associated with a disruption of normal anxiety-buffer functioning. A similar absence of the usual defensive suppression of death-related thoughts in response to mortality salience was found by Edmondson (2009). Whereas college students reporting low levels of trauma symptoms showed this suppression by not increasing death-thought accessibility in response to death reminders, those with moderate or high levels of symptoms responded to mortality salience with heightened death-thought accessibility. In a study with students of varying levels of trauma severity, Edmondson found that despite increased death-thought accessibility, students high in trauma severity did not engage in worldview defense following death reminders. Further, experimentally enhanced self-esteem, which has proven to be an effective buffer for non-traumatized individuals (e.g., Harmon-Jones et al., 1997), did not diminish the effects of death reminders on death-thought accessibility among these high trauma symptom participants.

The overall picture emerging from our work on trauma is that sudden dramatic confrontation with one's mortality can, in some instances, lead to a disruption of normal anxiety-buffer functioning. Such experiences leave the person overwhelmed with terror and, consequently, unable to function effectively or derive much pleasure from life. We find a markedly different pattern of coping among another group of people for whom death has become a more real and pressing concern—older adults.

COPING WITH DEATH IN LATER LIFE

Older adults are a unique population for understanding terror management processes. Although not terminally ill, this group is nearing the end of their lives and may have increasing medical problems and physical reminders of their increasing proximity to death. We wondered if their strategies for coping with death would differ from those of younger adults. At first glance, one might assume that older adults' greater temporal proximity to death and more frequent health problems would lead them to become even more vigilant in defending their worldviews and protecting their self-esteem. If mortality reminders lead younger adults to become increasingly defensive, shouldn't the more frequent and personally salient reminders of death associated with age lead older adults to be even more so? In addition, older adults' ability to live up to the mainstream cultural standards may have diminished, due to deterioration of physical and cognitive abilities that typically accompanies advancing age, resulting in decreased opportunity for building and maintaining self-esteem. Retirement, children moving away, and other changes in life circumstances further reduce their opportunities to feel valuable and needed. As time moves on and new generations take over the cultural mainstream, older adults' beliefs and values may no longer be as widely shared as they once were, undermining the validation for their worldviews that they enjoyed in their younger years. Further, the deaths of friends, family, and other people in their age group may decrease their opportunities for social interaction, undermining the protection they once received from relationships with others. In spite of—or, intriguingly, perhaps because of—what would appear to be significant obstacles preventing older adults from maintaining their anxiety-buffers, many older adults experience intact psychological health in later life, reporting higher levels of positive affect and lower levels of negative affect compared to younger adults (e.g., Lawton, Kleban, & Dean, 1993; Mroczek & Kolarz, 1998).

A family of psychological theories offers explanations for how older adults cope with the challenges of later life; these ideas might also help us understand what leads to better coping among the terminally ill. Baltes and Baltes (1990) proposed a model of selection optimization and compensation (SOC), which suggests that as people grow older, they select fewer activities to focus on, thus optimizing their skills and increasing their chances of success while compensating for the losses they may experience with age. In a similar vein, Heckhausen and Schulz's life span theory of control (1995) asserts that older adults increasingly rely on secondary control (i.e., control over their feelings about things that happen in their environment) as their ability to exert primary control (i.e., direct control over events in their environment) diminishes with age. The most widely researched theory of positive adaptation to aging is socioemotional selectivity theory, or SST (Carstensen, Isaacowitz, & Charles, 1999), which posits that perceived time limitations affect one's social and emotional goals. As people get older, their goals are increasingly aimed at having positive emotional experiences, compared to the seeking of a broader range of experiences, relationships, and information characteristic of young and middle adulthood. Although the theory initially focused on the effects of advancing age, related research identifies similar effects among the terminally ill. For example, Carstensen and Fredrickson (1998) found that among men with human immunodeficiency virus (HIV), differences were observed among those who were symptomatic and asymptomatic. More specifically, individuals with HIV-related symptoms possessed emotionally oriented social goals similar to older adults; they preferred to spend time with close friends and family members. This was interpreted as a means of maximizing positive emotional experiences when faced with time limitations. Individuals without HIV symptoms were found to maintain goals more similar to younger adults without HIV; they preferred to spend time networking with diverse social partners and acquaintances.

Consistent with this general picture of effective adaptation to the problems of advancing age, our own research has shown that older and younger adults differ considerably in how they respond to thoughts of death. Whereas mortality reminders lead younger adults to become more punitive toward individuals who have violated social norms, older adults become more lenient, suggesting a developmental shift toward a more flexible and perhaps forgiving strategy for maintaining psychological equanimity in the face of death (Maxfield et al., 2007). In a follow-up study (Maxfield, Pyszczynski, Greenberg, Pepin, & Davis, 2012), it was revealed that greater executive functioning (broadly defined as the cognitive abilities associated with complex planning, reasoning, and integration of information) predicted this pattern of increased leniency among older adults reminded of mortality; lesser executive functioning among older adults, on the other hand, was associated with increased punitiveness following a mortality reminder. For younger adults, the level of executive functioning did not impact responses to mortality. Memory functioning, self-reported health, and personal well-being did not predict how either older or younger adults responded to mortality reminders, suggesting that the specific resource of executive functioning may be required for older adults to be able to make the apparent transition to more flexible coping with their mortality. Because executive resources were predictive of only older adults' responses, it appears likely that the combination of accumulated life experience and retaining executive functioning abilities is essential for developing new ways of coping with more imminent mortality. We suspect that high levels of executive functioning are necessary for older adults to make the developmental transition to accommodate their new existential position in life—one in which death cannot be easily dismissed as something they can forestall until the distant and remote future.

It also appears that older adults adopt some unique ways of coping with their mortality that is particularly well-suited to their advanced age. As Erikson (1963), McAdams, de St. Aubin (1992), and many others have suggested, successful aging in general, and adaptation to increased proximity to death in particular, may entail letting go of egoistic pursuits and promotion of one's own individualized agendas and increased focus on the legacy they can pass on to others. In line with this possibility, we found older adults to express increased generative concern following a reminder of mortality, whereas younger adults' generativity was unaffected (Maxfield, Greenberg, Pyszczynski, Weise, & Kosloff, in press). In a second study, older adults responded to mortality with increased preference for creation of pro-social legacies involving positive contributions to society, with little attention to personal fame; this effect was not observed among younger adults.

Although in its beginning stages, research demonstrating transitions in how older adults cope with their increased temporal proximity to death might provide useful clues as to how some persons facing terminal diagnosis cope with their even greater proximity to death. Indeed, as suggested by Carstensen and Fredrickson's work (1998), some terminally ill persons may intuitively initiate similar shifts in strategies for adaptation and emotion regulation. Research demonstrating the devastating effects of disrupted anxiety-buffer functioning that sometimes accompanies traumatic experiences may also be relevant in that it informs us about processes involved in less successful coping with increased proximity to death. We now consider what these converging lines of theory and research might tell us about coping with terminal illness.

COPING WITH A TERMINAL DIAGNOSIS

It is hard to imagine a more distressing experience than being informed that you have an illness that is virtually certain to cause your death in a matter of months or years. We suspect that this is a scenario most people have imagined at some point in their lives (and that some imagine quite often), usually leading to a state of intense anxiety that quickly drives them to suppress these thoughts by diverting their attention to less distressing concerns. However, results are mixed regarding the psychological status of the seriously and terminally ill. One review reported depression rates ranging from a miniscule 1 percent to as high as 50 percent among individuals diagnosed with cancer (McDaniel, Musselman, Porter, Reed, & Nemeroff, 1995); these rates range from falling considerably short of to far exceeding the 8.7 percent rate of current depressive symptoms observed in the United States general population (15.7 percent lifetime depression; Strine et al., 2008). Similarly, although 11.3 percent of the U.S. population report meeting criteria for anxiety disorders at some point in their lifetime (Strine et al.), approximately 19.0 percent of individuals diagnosed with a range of cancer types meet criteria for an anxiety diagnosis, in addition to 22.6 percent of people diagnosed with cancer who report subclinical levels of anxiety (Linden, Vodermaier, MacKenzie, & Greig, in press).

Terminal diagnoses are also associated with PTSD, a particularly destabilizing set of reactions to extremely traumatic events usually involving threat to one's life that entails hyper-sensitivity to cues related to the trauma, intense anxiety and reactivity to threatening stimuli, recurring disruptive thoughts and images of the trauma, self-medication, numbing, and other behaviors aimed at avoiding such thoughts and feelings. In an overview of literature concerning reactions to a cancer diagnosis, 5 to 25 percent of patients meet diagnostic criteria for PTSD (Kangas, Henry, & Bryant, 2002). As many as 42 percent of women (Martinez, Israelski, Walker, & Koopman, 2002) and 30.2 percent of men (Kelly et al., 1998) meet diagnostic criteria for PTSD following a diagnosis of HIV.

Research on responses to terminal illness has included a wide range of types and stages of diseases, symptom severity, and surrounding life situations, which undoubtedly accounts for some of the variation in distress, coping, and adaptation. Nonetheless, this work clearly shows that diagnoses of a terminal illness present severe challenges to all who experience them and lead to overwhelming and debilitating psychological distress among many.

Related to these feelings of anxiety and depression, diagnosis of a terminal illness typically undermines people's assumptions about the world. Although we are all aware of the ever-present possibility of life-threatening disease and that many people suffer this fate every day, we tend to see ourselves as somehow immune, living in an imaginary world where such tragedy could not affect ourselves or those we love. Lerner (1980) referred to this belief in our invulnerability as a "fundamental delusion," born of our belief that the world is just, so bad things could not happen to good people like us. This is part of the reason that self-esteem protects us from anxiety: if we are good, we will not suffer. Consistent with these ideas, research has shown that most people are prone to underestimating the likelihood that negative events will occur in their lives and seem to assume that they are immune from disease (Weinstein, 1980). Because most, but not all, people harbor such illusions of personal invulnerability (hypochondriacs are an obvious exception), such beliefs are one reason that terminal diagnoses are unexpected and traumatic disconfirmations of core assumptions essential for maintaining psychological equanimity.

From the perspective of TMT, beliefs in one's invulnerability are central to the worldviews that protect people from a deeply rooted fear of death that results from an even more deeply rooted motive to continue living. Thus, fear of death is not a maladaptive or pathological response but rather an inherent and adaptive consequence of the desire for life. Human beings are designed by natural selection to respond with fear to anything that would end their lives. The terror management system was invented by our ancestors (quite unwittingly, of course) and then became part of the cultural knowledge that is transmitted over generations, through the socialization practices of parents and societies, to deal with the consequences of this desire for life among a species intelligent enough to realize that death is coming, even when there are no clear and present dangers of it. However, in the case of terminal illness, death is a clear and present danger. We suspect that realizing that fear and even terror have adaptive value might be helpful for some people facing such diseases in that it implies that their fears are indeed justified and appropriate and not evidence of weakness of character.

Although virtually everyone responds to terminal diagnoses with considerable fear and distress, some people cope with it much better than others. Starting with the pioneering work of Kübler-Ross (1969), many clinicians working with the dying have suggested that, for some, terminal illness provides an opportunity for psychological triumph. A growing body of research suggests that many individuals diagnosed with terminal illness report personal growth and positive shifts in perspective (for reviews of this literature, see Barskova & Oesterreich, 2009; Hefferon, Grealy, & Mutrie, 2009). Indeed, in her classic work concerning the stages of death and dying, Kübler-Ross (1969) described the responses to death, which, despite being initially characterized by denial, anger, bargaining and depression, can be followed by acceptance. Kübler-Ross specified, though, that this stage "should not be mistaken for a happy stage. It is almost void of feelings" (p. 124). However, more recent research seems to suggest that trauma may present opportunities for growth and a restructuring of one's life and priorities, a process which may indeed allow for a "happy stage" or improved psychological health. This process is referred to as posttraumatic growth, or PTG (Tedeschi & Calhoun, 1995), stress-related growth, and/or benefit finding.

Theories of PTG (e.g., Bonanno, 2004; Tedeschi & Calhoun, 2004) suggest that, because traumatic events violently challenge one's beliefs, sense of self, and relationships, they create opportunities for positive change and growth. PTG entails responding with improvement in at least some aspects of well-being, typically including things such as increased appreciation of life, changed priorities, closer relationships, enhanced feelings of personal strength, recognition of new possibilities, and spiritual development. Tedeschi and Calhoun (2004) argue that such positive growth in response to trauma is actually more common than serious dysfunction.

It is worth noting that there is considerable controversy as to whether such changes reflect actual changes in well-being or simply defensive distortions in the way people describe themselves to others and perhaps think about themselves privately as well (e.g., McFarland & Alvaro, 2000). It is well known that people often respond to threats by exaggerating their well-being and denying that they are bothered by their circumstances. For example, years ago we found that people respond to public failure with compensatory increases in privately assessed self-esteem (Greenberg & Pyszczynski, 1985). Although whether defensive denial is part of the process of PTG remains an important question, it may be that such shifts are helpful even if they do involve some level of self-deception. Clearly, greater understanding of the mechanisms involved in growth in response to trauma is needed.

Bringing these lines of theory and research together, the question becomes: what determines whether a person responds to terminal illness with fear, despair, and symptoms of PTSD, and what determines whether he or she instead adapts well and even exhibits improved well-being in response to illness? From the perspective of TMT, the question is: what leads to a collapse of the normal anxiety-buffering system, thus leading to extreme psychological distress; and on the other hand, what leads to the integration of the new challenges and ultimately leads to improved psychological organization that promotes increased openness, improved relationships, and greater appreciation of life?

We have recently argued that fear interferes with the ability to openly and objectively integrate new experiences into one's pre-existing worldview and often leads to both more biased integration of such information toward one's existing defensive strategies and general resistance to new information and experience (Pyszczynski, Greenberg, & Arndt, in press). Thus, we would expect that fearful responses to terminal diagnosis, which are probably almost universal in the early stages of coping, would at least initially inhibit growth and coping. The denial and anger observed by Kübler-Ross (1969) might be a reflection of this process. Problems with adjustment may be especially likely to become chronic when the initial response to the diagnosis involves dissociation, a tendency to psychologically withdraw in which one has an uncanny sense that what is happening is not real and sometimes feels like an outside observer of what is happening. Research has shown that dissociation is one of the strongest predictors of PTSD in response to trauma (e.g., Ozer et al., 2003) and that this link between dissociation and PTSD is mediated in part by a breakdown of normal anxiety-buffer functioning that persists long after the event (Abdollahi et al., 2011). We would expect that, generally speaking, the weaker their sense of meaning, self-worth, and interpersonal connectedness at the time, the less well people would cope with the traumatic diagnosis when they first receive it, the more likely such dissociation would occur, and the more likely they would experience long-term adverse consequences such as PTSD.

Interestingly, though, some research suggests that higher levels of distress prior to cancer treatments are actually predictive of greater PTG (e.g., Gallagher-Ross, 2012; Widows, Jacobsen, Booth-Jones, & Fields, 2005). This is consistent with Tedeschi and Calhoun's (2004) contention that traumatic distress can be an impetus to re-conceptualizing one's situation in a way that improves one's later well-being. Findings that reminders of death encourage greater structuring of information are also generally consistent with this idea (e.g., Landau et al., 2004). But when would higher levels of distress promote such positive reorganization of one's anxiety-buffering system and when would it lead to the system's collapse?

We suspect it may have much to do with whether one is able to control one's emotional responses so that they don't interfere with adaptive acceptance-promoting processing. Recent research suggests that mindfulness, a state associated with openly observing things as they happen without judging or evaluating or emphasis on their implications for one's own well-being may reduce the tendency to respond defensively to thoughts of one's mortality. Niemiec and colleagues (2010) reported that people high in mindfulness showed reduced levels of several different common worldview defenses in response to death reminders relative to persons lower in mindfulness. In a related vein, some studies have shown that a more open and in-depth confrontation with the idea of life's finality provokes greater attention to self-transcendent values and goals (Cozzolino, Staples, Meyers, & Samboceti, 2004; Lykins, Segerstrom, Averill, Evans, & Kemeny, 2007). There is some evidence that as death becomes more subjectively "real," people may become attuned to a more expansive and appreciative orientation to life (Cozzolino, Sheldon, Schachtman, & Meyers, 2009). Of course this begs the question of what might enable people to approach something as distressing, personally relevant, and potentially overwhelming as the news that they have a terminal illness. As has been suggested (e.g., Kübler-Ross, 1969), it may be that with something as devastating as terminal illness, people must first feel the full brunt of their situation and mourn their fate before they are able to step back and take the more mindful approach to their situation that would encourage acceptance and later growth.

The central point of the TMT analysis is that a strong well-functioning anxiety buffer makes it possible to respond to the threat by creatively integrating the threat and its implications into one's worldview and sense of self. Thus, people who, in the early stages of coming to terms with their disease, have high levels of meaning, purpose, self-esteem, and interpersonal connections should be able to adapt less defensively to their frightening situation. Studies showing that enhancing these psychological resources reduces death-thought accessibility and worldview defense are generally consistent with this possibility (for a review, see Pyszczynski & Kesebir, 2011). Research suggesting that PTG is most likely to occur among persons with high levels of meaning, spirituality (e.g., Smith, Dalen, Bernard, & Baumgartner, 2008), and social support (e.g., Barskova & Oesterreich, 2009) is also consistent with this possibility. This implies that helping patients maintain a sense of meaning, personal value, and relatedness should be an important goal for clinicians, caretakers, and loved ones as they process their diagnosis and its implications. This may be why social support is a good predictor of positive coping and PTG in response to severe illness (e.g., Scrignaro, Barni, & Magrin, 2010). The specifics of the prognosis and the likely impact and side effects of treatment are likely to also play an important role at this stage and influence the sorts of meanings and adaptations the person is able to make.

CLINICAL APPLICATIONS

From a terror management perspective, existential approaches to psychotherapy, like those advocated by Victor Frankl, R. D. Laing, Rollo May, Robert Jay Lifton, and Irvin Yalom will be most effective for working with the terminally ill. Working with the terminally ill to shore up their sense that, despite their physical maladies and limited life span, they are persons of value in a world of meaning with vital connections to friends and family—should have palliative consequences. And although there is currently a paucity of research evaluating the outcome of existential therapeutic approaches to treatment of the terminally ill, existing work is clearly in accord with this view.

William Breibart and colleagues developed a meaning-centered group psychotherapy, or MCGP (Breitbart, 2002; Greenstein & Breitbart, 2000) to help advanced cancer patients "sustain or enhance a sense of meaning, peace and purpose in their lives even as they approach the end of life" (Breibart et al., 2010, 23). The eight-week intervention, based on Viktor Frankl's work, employs traditional instruction, discussion, and experiential exercises. Each session explores different sources of meaning and significance (e.g., historical legacy; family legacy; accepting life's limitations; nature, art, and humor as sources of meaning; hopes for the future) and the impact of having cancer on one's sense of meaning and identity.

To determine the effectiveness of this intervention, Breibart et al. (2010) randomly assigned patients with advanced (stage III or IV) solid tumor cancers to either MCGP or a supportive group psychotherapy (SGP; focuses on encouraging patients to discuss concerns about their diagnosis and treatment, difficulties coping with cancer, and their experiences and emotions surrounding those experiences). Patients were assessed before and after completing the eight-week intervention, and two months thereafter. Spiritual well-being, meaning, hopelessness, desire for death, optimism/pessimism, anxiety, depression, and overall quality of life were assessed. MCGP produced significant improvements (over time and relative to SGP) in spiritual well-being and a sense of meaning, and treatment gains were more pronounced after two months. MCGP participants also reported decreased anxiety and desire for death, and these effects were also greater over time.

Breibart and colleagues cautioned that additional research is clearly in order to establish the magnitude and durability of these effects and to determine if MCGP is effective for people with different illnesses. However, these findings provide a strong empirical foundation in support of existentially based approaches to treating the terminally ill.

CONCLUSION AND FUTURE DIRECTIONS

For many, the terror associated with death is the uncertain. People are generally unaware of when they will die and how they will die; in fact, many suggest that the anxiety is associated with the knowledge that at any point, one's life could be ended by a random set of circumstances: being hit by a bus, dying in an airplane crash, or any number of other potentially lethal circumstances. However, for those who are acutely aware of their limited time and the factors which will likely cause their life's end, certainty may be of little comfort. With this unique awareness of life's fleeting nature and death's approach, individuals with terminal illness do appear to experience some depression and anxiety; however, many also experience personal growth. As we consider why some people are able to thrive as death approaches, research concerning how older adults and trauma survivors learn to cope may help us better understand areas where the terminally ill may struggle and opportunities for using some of the same strategies for developing more effective therapeutic interventions.

REFERENCES

Abdollahi, A., Pyszczynski, T., Maxfield, M., & Luszczynska, A. (2011). Posttraumatic stress reactions as a disruption in anxiety-buffer functioning: Dissociation and responses to mortality salience as predictors of severity of posttraumatic symptoms. *Psychological Trauma: Theory, Research, Practice, and Policy, 3*, 329–341.

American Psychiatric Association. (2000). Diagnostic and statistical manual of mental disorders (Revised 4th ed.). Washington, DC: APA.

Arndt, J., Greenberg, J., Solomon, S., Pyszczynski, T., & Simon, L. (1997). Suppression,accessibility of death-related thoughts, and cultural worldview defense: Exploring the psychodynamics of terror management. *Journal of Personality and Social Psychology, 73*, 5–18.

Arndt, J., Greenberg, J., Pyszczynski, T., & Solomon, S. (1997). Subliminal exposure to death-related stimuli increases defense of the cultural worldview. *Psychological Science, 8*, 379–385.

Arndt, J., Schimel, J., & Goldenberg, J. L. (2003). Death can be good for your health: Fitness intentions as a proximal and distal defense against mortality salience. *Journal of Applied Social Psychology, 33*, 1726–1746.

Baltes, P. B., & Baltes, M. M. (1990). Psychological perspectives on successful aging: The model of selective optimization and compensation. In P. B. Baltes & M. M. Baltes (Eds.), *Successful aging: Perspectives from behavioral sciences* (pp. 1–34). New York: Cambridge University Press.

Barskova, T., & Oesterreich, R. (2009). Posttraumatic growth in people living with a serious medical condition and its relations to physical and mental health: A systematic review. *Disability and Rehabilitation, 31*, 1709–1733.

Becker, E. (1973). *The denial of death*. New York: Free Press.

Benight, C. C., & Bandura, A. (2004). Social cognitive theory of posttraumatic recovery: The role of perceived self-efficacy. *Behaviour Research and Therapy, 42*, 1129–1148.

Bonanno, G. A. (2004). Loss, trauma, and human resilience: Have we underestimated the human capacity to thrive after extremely aversive events? *American Psychologist, 59*, 20–28.

Breitbart, W. (2002). Spirituality and meaning in supportive care: Spirituality and meaning-centered group psychotherapy intervention in advanced cancer. *Support Cancer Care, 10*, 272–280.

Breitbart, W., Rosenfeld, B., Gibson, C., Pessin, H., Poppito, S., Nelson, C., Tomarken, A., et al. (2010). Meaning-centered group psychotherapy for patients with advanced cancer: A pilot randomized controlled trial. *Psycho-Oncology, 19*, 21–28.

Carstensen, L. L., & Fredrickson, B. L. (1998). Influence of HIV status and age on cognitive representations of others. *Health Psychology, 17*, 494–503.

Carstensen, L. L., Isaacowitz, D. M., & Charles, S. T. (1999). Taking time seriously: A theory of socioemotional selectivity theory. *American Psychologist, 54*, 165–181.

Charles, S. T., & Carstensen, L. L. (2010). Social and emotional aging. *Annual Review of Psychology, 61*, 383–409.

Chatard, A., Pyszczynski, T., Arndt, J., Selimbegović, L., Konan, P. N., & Van der Linden, M. (2012). Extent of trauma exposure and PTSD symptom severity as predictors of anxiety-buffer functioning. *Psychological Trauma: Theory, Practice, Research, and Policy, 4,* 47–55.

Cozzolino, P. J., Sheldon, K. M., Schachtman, T. R., & Meyers, L. S. (2009). Limited time perspective, values, and greed: Imagining a limited future reduces avarice in extrinsic people. *Journal of Research in Personality, 43,* 399–408.

Cozzolino, P. J., Staples, A. D., Meyers, L. S., & Samboceti, J. (2004). Greed, death, and values: From terror management to transcendence management theory. *Personality and Social Psychology Bulletin, 30,* 278–292.

Edmondson, D. (2009). From shattered assumptions to weakened worldviews: Evidence of anxiety buffer disruption in individuals with trauma systems (Doctoral thesis). University of Connecticut.

Erikson, E. H. (1963). *Childhood and society.* New York: Norton.

Galea, S., Ahern, J., Resnick, H., Kilpatrick, D., Bucuvalas, M., Gold, J., et al. (2002). Psychological sequelae of the September 11 terrorist attacks in New York City. *New England Journal of Medicine, 346,* 982–987.

Gallagher-Ross, S. (2012). Predictors of posttraumatic growth in breast cancer survivors: An analysis of hardiness, attachment, and cognitive appraisal (Doctoral thesis). Fordham University.

Greenberg, J., Martens, A., Jonas, E., Eisenstadt, D., Pyszczynski, T., & Solomon, S. (2003). Psychological defense in anticipation of anxiety: Eliminating the potential for anxiety eliminates the effect of mortality salience on worldview defense. *Psychological Science, 14,* 516–519.

Greenberg, J., & Pyszczynski, T. (1985). Compensatory self-inflation: A response to threat to self-regard of public failure. *Journal of Personality and Social Psychology, 49,* 273–280.

Greenberg, J., Pyszczynski, T., & Solomon, S. (1986). The causes and consequences of a need for self-esteem: A terror management theory. In R. F. Baumeister (Ed.), *Public self and private self* (pp. 189–212). New York: SpringerVerlag.

Greenberg, J., Pyszczynski, T., Solomon, S., Pinel, E., Simon, L., & Jordan, K. (1993). Effects of self-esteem on vulnerability-denying defensive distortions: Further evidence of an anxiety-buffering function of self-esteem. *Journal of Experimental Social Psychology, 29,* 229–251.

Greenberg, J., Pyszczynski, T., Solomon, S., Rosenblatt, A., Veeder, M., Kirkland, S., & Lyon, D. (1990). Evidence for terror management theory II: The effects of mortality salience on reactions to those who threaten or bolster the cultural worldview. *Journal of Personality and Social Psychology, 58,* 308–318.

Greenberg, J., Simon, L., Harmon-Jones, E., Solomon, S., Pyszczynski, T., & Lyon, D. (1995). Testing alternative explanations for mortality salience effects: Terror management, value accessibility, or worrisome thoughts? *European Journal of Social Psychology, 25,* 417–433.

Greenberg, J., Solomon, S., & Arndt, J. (2008). A basic but uniquely human motivation: Terror management. In J. Shah & W. Gardner (Eds.). *Handbook of Motivation Science* (pp. 114–134). New York: Guilford Press.

Greenstein, M., & Breitbart, W. (2000). Cancer and the experience of meaning: A group psychotherapy program for people with cancer. *American Journal of Psychotherapy, 54,* 486–500.

Harmon-Jones, E., Simon, L., Greenberg, J., Pyszczynski, T., Solomon, S., & McGregor, H. A. (1997). Terror management theory and self-esteem: Evidence that increased self-esteem reduces mortality salience effects. *Journal of Personality and Social Psychology, 72,* 22–36.

Hayes, J., Schimel, J., Arndt, J., & Faucher, E. H. (2010). A theoretical and empirical review of the death thought accessibility concept in terror management research. *Psychological Bulletin, 136,* 699–739.

Heckhausen, J., & Schulz, R. (1995). A life-span theory of control. *Psychological Review, 102,* 284–304.

Hefferon, K., Grealy, M., & Mutrie, N. (2009). Posttraumatic growth and life-threatening physical illness: A systematic review of the qualitative literature. *British Journal of Health Psychology, 14,* 343–378.

James, W. (1950 [1890]). *The principles of psychology.* New York: Dover.

Janoff-Bulman, R. (1992). *Shattered assumptions: Towards a new psychology of trauma.* New York: Free Press.

Kangas, M., Henry, J. L., & Bryant, R. A. (2002). Posttraumatic stress disorder following cancer: A conceptual and empirical review. *Clinical Psychology Review, 22,* 499–524.

Kelly, B., Raphael, B., Judd, F., Perdices, M., Kernutt, G., Burnett, P., Dunne, M., & Burrows, G. (1998). Posttraumatic stress disorder in responses to HIV infection. *General Hospital Psychiatry, 20,* 345–352.

Kesebir, P., Luszczynska, A., Pyszczynski, T., & Benight, C. C. (2011). Posttraumatic stress disorder involves disrupted anxiety-buffer mechanisms. *Journal of Social and Clinical Psychology, 30,* 819–841.

Kübler-Ross, E. (1969). *On death and dying.* New York: Macmillan.

Landau, M. J., Johns, M., Greenberg, J., Pyszczynski, T., Martens, A., Goldenberg, J. L., et al. (2004). A function of form: Terror management and structuring the social world. *Journal of Personality and Social Psychology, 87,* 190–210.

Lawton, M. P., Kleban, M. H., & Dean, J. (1993). Affect and age: Cross-sectional comparisons of structure and prevalence. *Psychology and Aging, 8,* 165–175.

Lerner, M. J. (1980). *The belief in a just world: A fundamental delusion.* New York: Plenum Press.

Linden, W., Vodermaier, A., MacKenzie, R., & Greig, D. (in press). Anxiety and depression after cancer diagnosis: Prevalence rates by cancer type, gender, and age. *Journal of Affective Disorders.*

Lykins, E. L. B., Segerstrom, S. C., Averill, A. J., Evans, D. R., & Kemeny, M. E. (2007). Goal shifts following reminders of mortality: Reconciling posttraumatic growth and terror management theory. *Personality and Social Psychology Bulletin, 33,* 1088–1099.

Martinez, A., Israelski, D., Walker, C., & Koopman, C. (2002). Posttraumatic stress disorder in women attending human immunodeficiency virus outpatient clinics. *AIDS Patient Care and STDs, 16,* 283–291.

Maxfield, M., Greenberg, J., Pyszczynski, T., Weise, D., & Kosloff, S. (in press). *Evidence that reminders of mortality increase generative concern in older adults.*

Maxfield, M., Pyszczynski, T., Greenberg, J., Pepin, R., & Davis, H. P. (2012). The moderating role of executive functioning in older adults' responses to a reminder of mortality. *Psychology and Aging, 27,* 256–263.

Maxfield, M., Pyszczynski, T., Kluck, B., Cox, C., Greenberg, J., Solomon, S., & Weise, D. (2007). Age-related differences in responses to thoughts of one's own death: Mortality salience and judgments of moral transgressors. *Psychology and Aging, 22,* 343–351.

McAdams, D. P., & de St. Aubin, E. (1992). A theory of generativity and its assessment through self-report, behavioral acts, and narrative themes in autobiography. *Journal of Personality and Social Psychology, 62,* 1003–1015.

McDaniel, J. S., Musselman, D. L., Porter, M. R., Reed, D. A., & Nemeroff, C. B. (1995). Depression in patients with cancer: Diagnosis, biology, and treatment. *Archives of General Psychiatry, 52,* 89–99.

McFarland, C., & Alvaro, C. (2000). The impact of motivation on temporal comparisons: Coping with traumatic events by perceiving personal growth. *Journal of Personality and Social Psychology, 79,* 327–343.

Mikulincer, M., & Florian, V. (2002). The effects of mortality salience on self-serving attributions: Evidence for the function of self-esteem as a terror management mechanism. *Basic and Applied Social Psychology, 24,* 261–271.

Mikulincer, M., Florian, V., & Hirschberger, G. (2003). The existential function of close relationships: Introducing death into the science of love. *Personality and Social Psychology Review, 7,* 20–40.

Mroczek, D. K., & Kolarz, C. M. (1998). The effect of age on positive and negative affect: A developmental perspective on happiness. *Journal of Personality and Social Psychology, 75,* 1333–1349.

Niemiec, C. P., Brown, K. W., Kashdan, T. B., Cozzolino, P. J., Breen, W. E., Levesque-Bristol, C., & Ryan, R. M. (2010). Being present in the face of existential threat: The role of trait mindfulness in reducing defensive responses to mortality salience. *Journal of Personality and Social Psychology, 99,* 344–365.

Ozer, E. J., Best, S. R., Lipsey, T. L., & Weiss, D. S. (2003). Predictors of posttraumatic stress disorder and symptoms in adults: A meta-analysis. *Psychological Bulletin, 129,* 52–73.

Pyszczynski, T., Greenberg, J., & Arndt, J. (in press). Freedom vs. fear revisited. In M. Leary & J. Tangney, *Handbook of Self and Identity* (2nd ed.). New York: Guilford.

Pyszczynski, T., Greenberg, J., & Solomon, S. (1999). A dual process model of defense against conscious and unconscious death-related thoughts: An extension of terror management theory. *Psychological Review, 106,* 835–845.

Pyszczynski, T., & Kesebir, P. (2011). Anxiety buffer disruption theory: A terror management account of posttraumatic stress disorder. *Anxiety, Stress, & Coping, 24,* 3–26.

Rosenblatt, A., Greenberg., J., Solomon, S., Pyszczynski, T., & Lyon, D. (1989). Evidence for terror management theory I: The effects of mortality salience on reactions to those who violate or uphold cultural values. *Journal of Personality and Social Psychology, 57,* 681–690.

Routledge, C., Arndt, J., & Goldenberg, J. L. (2004). A time to tan: Proximal and distal effects of mortality salience on sun exposure intentions. *Personality and Social Psychology Bulletin, 30,* 1347–1358.

Schimel, J., Hayes, J., Williams, T., & Jahrig, J. (2007). Is death really the worm at the core? Converging evidence that worldview threat increases death-thought accessibility. *Journal of Personality and Social Psychology, 92,* 789–803.

Scrignaro, M., Barni, S., & Magrin, M. E. (2010). The combined contribution of social support and coping strategies in predicting post-traumatic growth: A longitudinal study on cancer patients. *Psycho-Oncology, 20,* 823–831.

Silver, R. C., Holman, E. A., McIntosh, D. N., Poulin, M., & Gil-Rivas, V. (2002). Nationwide longitudinal study of psychological responses to September 11. *Journal of the American Medical Association, 288,* 1235–1244.

Smith, B. W., Dalen, J., Bernard, J. F., & Baumgartner, K. B. (2008). Posttraumatic growth in non-Hispanic white and Hispanic women with cervical cancer. *Journal of Psychosocial Oncology, 26,* 91–109.

Solomon, S., Greenberg, J., & Pyszczynski, T. (1991). A terror management theory of social behavior: The psychological functions of self-esteem and cultural worldviews. In M. Zanna (Ed.), *Advances in experimental social psychology* (Vol. 24, pp. 91–159). Orlando, FL: Academic Press.

———. (1998). Tales from the crypt: On the role of death in life. *Zygon, 33*(1), 9–43.

Strachan, E., Schimel, J., Arndt, J., Williams, T., Solomon, S., Pyszczynski, T., & Greenberg, J. (2007). Terror mismanagement: Evidence that mortality salience exacerbates phobic and compulsive behaviors. *Personality and Social Psychology Bulletin, 33,* 1137–1151.

Strine, T. W., Mokdad, A. H., Balluz, L. S., Gonzalez, O., Crider, R., Berry, J. T., & Kroenke, K. (2008). Depression and anxiety in the United States: Findings from the 2006 Behavioral Risk Factor Surveillance System. *Psychiatric Services, 59,* 1383–1390.

Tedeschi, R. G., & Calhoun, L. G. (1995). *Trauma and transformation: Growing in the Aftermath of suffering.* Thousand Oaks, CA: Sage.

———. (2004). Posttraumatic growth: Conceptual foundations and empirical evidence. *Psychological Inquiry, 15,* 1–8.

Tedstone, J. E., & Tarrier, N. (2003). Posttraumatic stress disorder following medical illness and treatment. *Clinical Psychology Review, 23,* 409–448.

Weinstein, N. D. (1980). Unrealistic optimism about future life events. *Journal of Personality and Social Psychology, 39,* 806–820.

Widows, M. R., Jacobsen, P. B., Booth-Jones, M., & Fields, K. K. (2005). Predictors of posttraumatic growth following bone marrow transplantation for cancer. *Health Psychology, 24,* 266–273.

Chapter Six

Psychoanalytic Literature on the Treatments of Dying Patients

Norman Straker, MD

There are relatively few published papers by psychoanalysts that discuss the treatment of patients facing death. In general, the published papers tend to fall into three main categories. The earliest case reports are by Eissler, Norton, and Roose. They were a major departure from standard psychoanalytic technique. They stressed the need for an approach that was specifically designed for dying patients. More recent papers have tended to fall into two major categories, depending on where they are published. Mainstream psychoanalytic journals have limited their publications to only those cases that fit the classical paradigm. They have also published multiple reports of the impact of serious illness in psychoanalysts and how psychoanalytic technique should be altered to deal with the analysts' illnesses. These classical papers report that patients who developed terminal cancer during their analysis could continue in a classical analysis with minimal modifications. Other journals and books report on treatments that are more flexible in approach and overlap with psychoanalytic psychotherapy. The need for the analyst to be more responsive to the patient's unique situation is highlighted in these less classical case descriptions.

Eissler, Norton, and Roose wrote the earliest classical psychoanalytic papers on the treatment of dying patients more than forty years ago. Their contributions were a major departure from orthodox technique and highly responsive to the patient's life crisis. Their papers were our guides for the psychotherapeutic treatment of cancer patients when I began my work in 1976 at Memorial Sloan-Kettering.

Eissler, in his book *The Psychiatrist and the Dying Patient*, was the first to stress the unique role that the psychiatrist or psychoanalyst could offer dying patients (Eissler, 1955). In contrast to the orthodox technique, which places interpretation at the center of psychoanalytic therapy, he demonstrated an activist approach in each of his three cases. He recommended a relationship "without limits" for the treatment of dying cancer patients. He described giving his patients "sublimated love" to try to recreate the early mother-child relationship. He stressed the importance of having an attitude of "sorrow and pity" and a belief in the immortality of his patient. He termed his approach a "gift situation." Using this approach, the psychoanalyst creates an experience where the patient feels they are dying together.

In *The Treatment of the Dying Patient* (1963) Norton described the treatment of a women with cancer, referred to her because of a desire to commit suicide. Norton learned that her desire for suicide was preceded by an abandonment by her minister. He had withdrawn from her during their philosophical discussions about death. Norton recognized the abandonment by the minister repeated the patient's childhood fears of abandonment. She instituted daily visits and made herself totally available to the patient.

As the patient's health deteriorated, Norton described various stages of the patient's regression. The first regression occurred after Norton gave the patient permission to "be a baby." A second stage of regression occurred after the patient lost her sight from a brain metastasis. In the final stage of regression, "introjection," the patient described the feeling that the therapist was with her twenty-four hours a day. The blurring of boundaries and the merging fantasy were protective of pain, isolation, and aloneness. At times, the patient was noted to call the therapist "Mother." In her discussion, Norton concluded that the "gift situation," as described by Eissler, was best understood as the establishment of the regressive transference.

Roose described a physician patient referred to him as a suicidal risk (1969). The physician patient had told his doctor that he would kill himself if he had a confirmed cancer diagnosis. His doctor told him that he had a granuloma, not cancer. The patient could speak about his fears of dying and his concerns about being provided with a proper burial only with the psychoanalyst. Roose challenged the patient to live up to his high life ideals as a counter to his desires for suicide. As the patient entered the last phases of the disease, the author noted that denial and regression helped the patient became convinced of his own immortality.

As I noted in my introduction, these three papers gave those of us at Sloan-Kettering Cancer Center an approach to the psychoanalytic treatment of cancer patients in the earliest years of the development of psycho-oncology. Their papers gave permission to move away from the psychotherapy practice of the time—passive listening and interventions that were primarily interpretations of genetic or transference material. These three analysts recognized that facing death was an existential crisis that required a different technique than was in vogue for neurotic or psychotic patients at that time.

Their technique, however, was a product of the time, a time when cancer was considered a death sentence and the course of the illness was, in most cases, a journey from diagnosis to death with little hope of a cure or a long survival. There was also no palliative or hospice care, and the psychiatrist or psychoanalyst was often the only professional who accompanied the patient from diagnosis to death. Therefore, in each of these cases the emphasis was on encouraging a regressive transference as the best protection near the end of life against anxiety and pain to help the patient have a peaceful death.

As the treatments of cancer became more effective, the course of the disease has become much more attenuated, uncertain, and unpredictable. Also, palliative and hospice care are now available to patients whose active treatments are no longer effective. Concurrent with these changes, I have proposed changes in how psychoanalysts treat patients. An approach emerges that combines the value of analytic listening, interpretation, transference, countertransference focus, existential psychoanalytic psychotherapy, and an activist agenda that meets the requirements of the crisis of facing death, while pursing emotional growth and meaning. A detailed account of my recommendations follows a review of the literature. This is a chronological review of the publications from psychoanalytic electronic publications. It addresses analytic case reports, observations of defenses, powerful countertransference, and different aspects of the psychoanalytic treatment that is unique to the treatment of dying patients.

Hagglund offers a construct that is used by dying patients to deal with the narcissistic conflict between the patient's weak and ailing body and the wished-for ideal state.

> He creates a fantasy of his own body as a cleansed or better form . . . in which the body-self attains a libidinal value. Such a fantasy can be of going to heaven or returning to a flawless state or a mental-self or survival through one's own children, achievements, and the mental images achieved in other's minds. The splitting in the dying person's mind allows for the mourning of the body and the cathexis is shifted to the fantasy world and the transference to the analyst. This is otherwise known as transcendence, in the face of death. The last adaptive attempt at maturation in the mourning process of the dying person is the integration of the essential phases of his life and his relationships and the desire to share his concrete created product with others, as a gift, transferring one's narcissism so it will live on. The desire to connect to loved ones, talk about one's experience and hold on to the objects of the world is an attempt to cling to life. (Hagglund, 1981)

Tasman notes that the dying patient may need the psychoanalyst to function as a self-object who takes over the functions of self-regulation or serves as an idealized all-powerful protector. While this report was presented to deal with a patient responding to terminal illness as a severe narcissistic injury, using a

self-object model from Kohut (1977), I have personally found that the analyst might consider functioning as a self-object for patients suffering from
brain cancer or some degree of mental impairment (Tasman, 1982).

MORE RECENT PAPERS

Minerbo makes a strong argument for the treatment of all dying cancer
patients using an orthodox approach. He initially "felt unsure that he could
personally deal with this tragic situation without deviating from an analytic
stance." In fact, the author reported several interpretations to the patient that
challenged her attempt to deny her imminent death. The patient, attempting
to find some comfort in denial, was reported to have said, "You are the
analyst to the end." Minerbo says he agrees with Bail (1981) "that colluding
with the patient's negation of death is deceitful and destroys what is most
courageous in man." In my view, permitting some denial does not deprive
the patient of the truth nor is it being deceptive. Terminally ill patients deny
and face their death intermittently and continuously as part of successful
coping. This analyst's devotion to "truth" and the decision to "not collude
with denial" has the feel, to me, of cruelty. It is a failure to put the needs of a
dying patient, who very clearly understands her precarious state, before an
inflexible adherence to technique. This same patient requested that her analyst see the patient's daughter after she died so as to have some sense of
continuity with the analyst after her death. He is reported to have replied that
he could see her but never treat. Once again, he seemed, to me, to put
adherence to technique before a simple uncomplicated response that would
give a dying patient some solace. This author's "non-psychoanalytic stance,"
presented apologetically, (p. 86) "that perhaps what she should do was make
the best possible use of the time she had left," seemed to have been very
helpful. His concluding remarks reject any modifications in technique as
undercutting the value of analysis. This conclusion is based on the treatment
of just this one patient whose analysis was continued in the terminal phase
over the telephone (Minerbo, 1998).

Mayer describes "being ruthless, inspirational, and compassionate" in
response to her patient's limited life span in a case report (Mayer, 1994). She
modified her technique and became much more assertive about the issues
that the analyst felt needed to be resolved to complete the analysis. At times
the analyst seemed confident in suggesting to the patient that the "patient's
focus on dying was a resistance to a complete analysis of the transference."
The patient argued with the analyst, saying the analyst had no idea of what it
was like to be dying. Despite this the analyst persisted.

While the analyst's interpretation may have been correct, it raises the
possibility, for me, that the patient's needed focus on her impending death

just made the analyst so uncomfortable that the analyst directed their attention to the transference. In this report, a termination date was set and met one month before the patient died. The assertive technique and planned termination during the time of the patient's impending death has the feel of a denial of the finality of death and a planned avoidance of witnessing the patient's last days by the analyst. More recent reports tend to be more sensitive to the needs of this unique life situation and less preoccupied with proving that a classical stance is viable.

Adams-Silvan writes about her conflict with abandoning her usual technique in the best interest of helping her dying patient. She describes a very thoughtful supportive psychoanalytic treatment that is initially modified to help the patient to find the strength to fight her terminal illness until the patient decides to take her own life. The analyst's acceptance of the patient's decision allowed her to find a peaceful end to her nightmare. This report demonstrates how an experienced, flexible psychoanalyst can ease the suffering of a patient with limited psychological resources by using psychoanalytic listening. Her flexible approach "brought a sense of control that calmed the patient's terror of dying, that could not be achieved by an in depth psychoanalysis." Her paper is reproduced in this book (chapter 8) and is an important contribution to facing death (Adams-Silvan, 1994).

Bustamante's (2001) view is more in line with mine. "When a trained analyst is available, analysis can take place but not in the orthodox sense, particularly if the patient is in the advanced stages of illness. What can be done, however, is analytic listening and work with illness, death and mourning. It is important to clarify whether the patient is a suitable subject for psychotherapy or psychoanalytic intervention." The author recommends for the patient "hope in the form of the desire, not to suffer pain in the dying, to hear that the closest relatives have accepted the patient's impending death, to see and say good-bye to the most important persons in their life, to finally attain rest and a better life beyond death."

Berzoff (2004) notes that doing psychotherapy with a dying patient may call for abandoning neutrality, for bending the analytic frame for facing one's own mortality, and for tolerating the chaotic and unpredictable nature of the course of an illness.

Rodin and Zimmerman (2008) note that when one is confronted with one's mortality it triggers a search for meaning and results in opportunities for emotional growth. They also point out that "death anxiety" in the physically healthy person may not have the same meaning or significance as it does in the terminally ill. They note that there is growing evidence that seriously ill patients and their families tend to favor honesty and directness in communication of prognostic information and preparation for the end of life (Kirk, Kirk, & Kristjanson, 2004) in contrast to the general population who tend to want to deny death anxiety (Rank, 1958; Becker, 1973; Langs, 2003).

These new observations suggest that the static concept of "denial of death" underestimates the multiple fluctuating and variable integrations of one's experience.

My observations support the view that the "awareness of death" and the acceptance of one's mortality is compatible with a desire to live and does not have to be associated with depression and demoralization because self-experience about these matters are fluid, shifting, and multiple (Mitchell, 1993). Compatible with this view is that "dissociation . . . may be a fundamental defense mechanism and that subjective experiences are composed of multiple and shifting self-states and self-organizations generated in societal and interpersonal fields" (Mitchell, 1997). In fact, Mitchell (2002) suggests that mental health may be understood in terms of the capacity to sustain and tolerate such discontinuous self-states. This view is compatible with individuals "double awareness" of a foreshortened life or even imminent death, coexisting with a strong will to live and a tendency to find meaning (Rodin et al., 2007). It is probable that the capacity to simultaneously hold the idea of living and dying is the most important psychological task for those who are facing death. Suicidality or a desire for hastened death may be regarded as a failure to sustain this duality of thinking. Erikson (1982) promoted the view that facing death anxiety can promote the developmental stage of integrity versus despair to the final stage of generativity. This view is compatible with the view of Frankl (1963). The challenge of authentic self-awareness in the face of mortality depends on the individual's capacity to tolerate the ongoing dialectic of different self-states (Bromberg, 1998).

Attachment theory also makes a contribution to our observations and treatment of dying patients. Death anxiety is diminished in those with secure attachments and may enhance the capacity to process painful affect states and face the end of life without a loss of hope and meaning. Psychotherapeutic approaches that address and allow for a renegotiation of attachment relationships in light of illness are important. Those who have "insecure attachments" or those who are highly self-reliant need to enhance their attachment security buffer against depression and demoralization (Florian, Mikulincer, & Hischberger, 2002).

Daehnert's paper "Crossing Over: A Story of Surrender and Transformation" (2008) is a poignant account of a psychoanalyst's treatment of a dying patient. In it she describes the creative process that occurs when an analyst engages with a terminally ill patient. In contrast to those who attempt to uphold a more orthodox stance, she permits herself to "expand the boundaries of her relationship to create a rhythm together that carried the patient into death." In my view, she demonstrates the richness of an encounter with a dying patient when a psychoanalyst can be flexible and permit the evolution of a meaningful, creative "shared mental space that is based on a mix of transference, countertransference, as well as the analyst as a new authentic object who can be known as required by the situation. The acknowledgement by the analyst that the dying patient's impending death is meaningful and their experience together will live on is validating and necessary to helping the patient surrender." The author attributes this awareness to Ghent (1990): "Surrender for Ghent involved a deep yearning to be known, to live completely in the present and have a chance for personal transformation by letting go in the presence of another." The author also permits her patient access to her own dreams as she expands her boundaries in the service of helping her patient experience the joint impact of the dying experience. Finally, the author acknowledges that the paper is "my art of mourning, is my attempt to reclaim my separateness and do justice to the complexity and intensity of my experience with loss. It is my gift and my return." The patient lives on through the story and in the analyst (Daehnert, 2008).

Finally, I recommend the work of Breitbart, a colleague of mine and a non-psychoanalyst who has developed meaning-centered group psychotherapy for terminally ill patients. His therapy, based on Frankl's logotherapy, helps patients avoid demoralization and a desire for hastened death (Breitbart et al., 2000). It is instructive for psychoanalysts as it demonstrates the necessity and empirical effectiveness of incorporating existential issues in their treatment of dying patients.

REFERENCES

Adams-Silvan, A. (1994). That darkness is about to pass: The treatment of a dying patient. *The Psychoanalytic Study of the Child, 49*, 328–348.

Bail, B. (1981). To practice one's art. In J. S. Grotstein (Ed.), *Do I Dare Disturb the Universe? A Memorial to W. R. Bion's Beverly Hills*. London: Caesura Press, 59–81.

Becker, E. (1973). *The denial of death*. New York: Free Press.

Berzoff, J. (2004). When a client dies, a commentary. *Psychoanalytic Social Work, 11*, 15–22.

Breitbart, W., Rosenfeld, B., Pessin, H., Kim, M., Funesti-Esch, J., Galietta, M., Nelson, C. J., & Brescia, R. (2000). Depression, hopelessness, and desire for hastened death in terminally ill patients with cancer. *Journal of the American Medical Association, 284*, 2907–2911.

Bromberg, P. (1998). *Standing in the spaces: Essays on clinical process, trauma, and dissociation*. Hillsdale, NJ: Analytic Press.

Bustamante, J. J. (2001). Understanding hope in the process of dying. *International Forum Psychanal, 10*, 49–55.

Daehnert, C. (2008). Crossing over: A story of surrender and transformation. *Contemporary Psychoanalysis, 44*, 199–218.

Eissler, K. (1955). *The psychiatrist and the dying patient*. New York: International University Press.

Erikson, E. H. (1982). *The life cycle completed: A review*. New York: Norton.

Florian, V., Mikulincer, M., & Hirschberger, G. (2002). The anxiety-buffering function of close relationships: Evidence that relationship commitment acts as a terror management mechanism. *Journal of Personality and Social Psychology, 82*, 527–542.

Frankl, V. (1963). *Man's search for meaning*. Boston: Beacon Press.

Ghent, E. (1990). Masochism, submission, surrender. *Contemporary Psychoanalysis, 26*, 108–135.

Hagglund, T. B. (1981). The final stages of the dying process. *International Journal of Psychoanalysis, 62*, 45–49.

Hoffman, I. Z. (1998). Death, anxiety, and adaptation to mortality in psychoanalytic theory. *Ritual and spontaneity in the psychoanalytic process.* Hillsdale, NJ: The Analytic Press, 31–67.

Kirk, P., Kirk, I., & Kristjanson, L. J. (2004). What do patients receiving palliative care for cancer and their families want to be told? A Canadian and Australian qualitative study. *British Medical Journal, 328*, 1343.

Kohut, H. (1977). *Restoration of the self.* New York: International Universities Press.

Langs, R. (1997). *Death, anxiety, and clinical practice.* London: Karnac Books.

———. (2003). Adaptive insights into death anxiety. *Psychoanalytic Review, 90*, 565

Mayer, E. L. (1994). Some implications for psychoanalytic technique drawn from analysis of a dying patient. *Psychoanalytic Quarterly, 63*, 1.

Minerbo, V. (1998). The patient without a couch: An analysis of a patient with terminal cancer.*International Journal of Psychoanalysis, 79*, 83.

Mitchell, S. (1993). *Hope and dread in psychoanalysis.* New York: Basic Books.

———. (1997). *Influence and autonomy in psychoanalysis.* Hillsdale, NJ: Analytic Press.

———. (2002). The treatment of choice: A response to Susan Fairfield. In S. Fairfield, L. Layton, & C. Stack (Eds.), *Bringing the plague: Toward a postmodern psychoanalysis* (pp. 103–111). New York: Other Press.

Norton, J. (1963). The treatment of a dying patient. *The Psychoanalytic Study of the Child, 18*, 541.

Rank, O. (1958). *Beyond psychology.* New York: Dover Publications.

Rodin, G., & Gillies, L. A. (2000). Individual psychotherapy for the patient with advanced disease. In H. M. Chochinov & W. Breitbart (Eds.), *Handbook of Psychiatry in Palliative Medicine* (pp. 189–196). New York: Oxford University Press.

Rodin, G., Walsh, A., Zimmermann, C., Gagliese, L., Jones, J., Shepherd, F. A., Moore, M., Braun, M., Donner, A., & Mikulincer, M. (2007). The contribution of attachment security and social support to depressive symptoms in patients with metastatic cancer. *Psycho-Oncology, 16*, 1080–1097.

Rodin, G., Zimmermann, C., Rydall, A., Jones, J., Shepherd, F.A., Moore M., Fruh, M., Donner, A., & Gagliese, L. (2007). The desire for hastened death in patients with metastatic cancer. *Journal of Pain and Symptom Management, 33*, 661.

Rodin, G., & Zimmermann, C. (2008). Psychoanalytic reflections on mortality: A reconsideration. *Journal of the American Academy of Psychoanalysis and Dynamic Psychiatry, 36*, 181–196.

Roose, L. (1969). The dying patient. *The International Journal of Psychoanalysis, 50*(3), 385–397.

Tasman, A. (1982). Loss of self-cohesion in terminal illness. *Journal of the Academy of Psychoanalysis and Dynamic Psychiatry, 10*, 515–526.

Chapter Seven

An Update in the Psychoanalytic Treatment of the Cancer Patient Facing Death

Norman Straker, MD

My first recommendation for the psychoanalyst engaged in the treatment of cancer patients facing death is for them to have a flexible approach. This point is also made in the Adams-Silvan, Barnhill, Luber, Philips, and Plopa chapters as well as in most papers in my review of the literature. The patient is engaged, and responded to, based on who they are, where they are in their illness, and what they present in the session to the analyst. The two papers published in mainstream psychoanalytic journals portray case reports of treatments to demonstrate that a strict analytic stance is both possible and worthwhile. These reports that I reviewed earlier attempted to make the case for the appropriateness and usefulness of continuing an orthodox analysis with few modifications in a patient who is dying (Mayer, 1994; Minerbo, 1998). In one case the patient was told that her focus on dying was a resistance to the analysis of the transference. Although this interpretation may have been true, it also seems to suggest a retreat to orthodoxy from the death anxiety aroused in the analyst. This patient's analysis was terminated one month prior to her death. While this achievement was seen as a triumph, it is contrary to the most enduring principle of palliative care that views caring attachments as buffers for the patient in the face of imminent death.

In the other case, the analyst frequently focuses on interpreting the patient's denial of impending death as a search for truth. As noted in the review chapter, it is well established that dying patients vacillate in their attention to their nearness to death as a way to best live out their dying days. The truth is not lost on those who are close to death, and reminding patients of that fact is not necessarily helpful to the treatment. In contrast to this approach, I recommend a commonsense approach to denial in the later part of this update chapter. These two classical psychoanalytic cases were ongoing when cancer appeared during the analysis. They are contrasted with the reports that are predominant in the literature and in this book.

This flexibility and active approach, first described by Eissler (1955), Norton (1963), and Roose (1969), which were in complete contrast to ongoing analytic practice of that time, can now be integrated with psychoanalytic listening and interventions if the patient is capable psychologically and physically. While each individual treatment will unfold in its own unique manner, consideration should be given to the inclusion of the recommendations that will promote the most adaptive strategies for the analyst and patient facing death (Straker, 1990, 1998, 2008). Some analysts continue with the earliest views of Freud—that the fear of death does not exist in the unconscious mind but is only a derivative of the conflicts of childhood. This view suggests that the analysis of the fears of childhood will lessen death anxiety. This is not the view of this author. Death anxiety is not only unconsciously present (clinically and empirically), as demonstrated in earlier chapters, but it is also intermittently present in consciousness where it cannot be denied. Therefore, patients with cancer who experience conscious death anxiety need to be engaged in facing their mortality rather than avoiding the issue. If that happens, the analysts will be abandoning the patients to their own private fears.

THE PSYCHOANALYST NEEDS TO BE
AWARE OF SURVIVAL TIME ISSUES

Earlier in the book I wrote about the oncologist's anxiety facing death, especially at the time that it becomes apparent that the oncological treatment will not bring about a cure. I noted that the oncologist's poorly managed anxiety could lead to two problematic outcomes. One is the continuation of aggressive cancer therapies that are futile and do not address suffering. The other can be an off-handed blunt, anxious, blurted-out prognosis of the time of death without an allotment of time to help the patient and family process the information. This survival time proclamation can feel like a God-like pronouncement. While the seemingly accurate prognosis may restore the self-esteem of the oncologist for loss of the battle against cancer, it is emotionally problematic. Regardless of its motivation, it is received by his patient and family as a firm date and experienced as "a death sentence" with obvious psychological consequences.

I have had a number of referrals for psychoanalytic psychotherapy that have followed statements like "You have three months to live. There is nothing we can do." Such a proclamation that does not make clear that these predictions are best guesses based on averages, and are often out of date and can result in demoralization and in a loss of quality of living time. My experiences with these less than humble pronouncements, which are usually inaccurate, have changed my approach to the treatment of all cancer patients who are facing death and have been given a poor prognosis.

I now prefer to have patients with illnesses that have no cure think of themselves as "patients living with uncertainty." When I began my work, I too accepted these pronouncements as accurate; however, I reserve the designation of being a "dying patient" to a time when the patient is actually dying. This approach does not deny the inevitability of death; rather, it attempts to maximize the remaining healthy time without a loss of hope. It permits the patient to keep a positive focus on life to the extent that that is possible while one is alive. My approach is in harmony with Stephen Jay Gould, who wrote *The Median Isn't the Message* (1985) after he was diagnosed with mesothelioma. His median survival time after diagnosis was six months. Being a naturalist, he researched the patient-survival curves and took solace in the finding that patients with mesothelioma failed to cluster around the median survival time. He lived twenty years after the surgery and chemotherapy. I am also in agreement with a recent study published in *Cancer* that concludes that the majority of doctors prefer to wait until health declines before initiating discussions that predict six months left to live so that end-of-life options can be offered (Keating et al., 2010).

The video "The Courage to Survive" (Straker, website 2005) which is available for viewing on the psychoanalytic blog under "Video," demonstrates the negative impact of an incorrect prediction of survival time. In this video, the patient was given a three-month survival time. The husband and patient then experienced each day as one day less to live rather than focusing on quality of life. This patient lived for several years beyond the three-month prediction. Two other patients I have treated were also given survival time pronouncements which they experienced as death sentences. In one situation, the diagnosis was incorrect; in the other, a more thoughtful, careful explanation of the inability to predict outcome would have saved my patient great psychological pain.

Case 1

A seventy-six-year-old married woman was told on the telephone by her internist of more than thirty years, "You have final stage lung cancer, and you need to go immediately to Sloan-Kettering Cancer Center." Two months later, she was rediagnosed with stage III lymphoma with lung infiltrates. Her oncologist referred her to me after she began responding to the chemotherapy. She had retreated from all her usual activities in preparation for her death. Despite the medical improvement she persisted in the belief that she was dying.

When we first met she did not agree with me that she would survive. She did agree, however, that she was very anxious and depressed and accepted my recommendation for weekly psychotherapy visits and an antidepressant. After seeing her much improved recent scans and comparing them with her first diagnostic scans, she was ready to accept my suggestion that she now might try to think of herself as a person who was living with uncertainty. She agreed and our therapeutic work could now focus on mobilizing her to return to her former life activities. After the second phase of the chemotherapy, her scans revealed that she was in complete remission. She returned to church and resumed all former activities. She was discharged from psychiatric treatment with an optimistic feeling that she had many days in front of her.

Case 2

A sixty-four-year-old married writer discovered accidentally on a MRI that she had early lung cancer non-small cell type. The first infiltrates were surgically removed and she was given a very favorable prognosis. A follow-up MRI six months later revealed a second lesion. She was now told "that if these infiltrates were malignant, you will be dead within the year."

She came to see me shortly after her new prognosis. She was prepared to die within the year. She was very depressed and had panic attacks. She requested that I help her complete a novel that would familiarize her grandchildren with her family before she died. We began a twice-weekly psychoanalytic psychotherapy and antidepressants.

I felt she would have more energy to write if she could accept her situation as uncertain rather than as a death sentence. I proposed that we explore why she had taken the view that death was imminent when she had, in fact, an uncertain prognosis. Her early history provided some important clues as to why she was reluctant to be open to uncertainty. My patient had a longstanding desire to be sick like her sister, who died when she was just thirteen years old of chronic renal disease.

A longstanding estrangement with her daughter and her three grandchildren motivated the book project. The book was to be the connection with the grandchildren who she had lost. I learned that my patient unconsciously treated her own daughter in childhood as she would have wanted to treat her sick sibling. She was harsh, critical, and not indulgent. An early divorce created further hostility with her daughter, who saw her father as her mother's victim. She emerged as a rebelliousness angry adolescent who was never close to her mother. My patient, as a result of her exploratory therapy, acknowledged her critical and hostile attitude toward her daughter. She asked for forgiveness and a chance to be a better mother before she died. These dialogues allowed for some reconciliation, visits, and travel with the grandchildren.

The MRI showed no change at the end of the year, which indicated that the lesions were not malignant. The patient continued to believe she was dying. The therapeutic challenge was her difficulty giving up the long desired sick role. She eventually recognized that being sick was not as desirable as she might have thought during her childhood. It also represented a punishment for her guilty feelings. The opportunity now existed to not only reconnect with her daughter but also to enjoy the relationships with her three grandchildren. She accepted the idea that she could try to live with uncertainty. Fully recovered from her depression, she returned to her former career and visited her daughter and grandchildren frequently. Her health is now stable; she is no longer depressed and is cancer-free four years later.

"A RELATIONSHIP WITHOUT LIMITS" (EISSLER) IS NO LONGER NECESSARY

My treatment approach evolved over a thirty-five-year period. I have treated at least twenty cancer patients until their death and supervised countless fellows who have cared for dying patients. In the late 1970s, when I began this work, I would see the patients almost daily in the hospital or at their home (per Eissler). I believed that this was the best method to facilitate the regressive transference, which would promote the most peaceful death. When the patients were dying at home, my role was often both psychological and medical, especially if there was no medical coverage. I worked in isolation, as the care of dying patients was not as yet a specialty.

More recently, specialists in pain management, palliative, and hospice care have become available. Advance directives and DNR discussions are now routine by the oncologist, in contrast to the past when the psychoanalyst may have been the first to talk with the patient about facing death. As a result of all these changes, I no longer function in isolation. I am now part of a team that includes palliative and hospice care. The palliative care and hospice staff provides good pain control, emotional support, and comfort care, in contrast to the past when all these functions fell to me. Therefore, with daily comfort care reassigned, the psychoanalytic relationship without limits (Eissler) with daily visits is no longer necessary. I can now focus more exclusively on the emotional issues facing dying patients.

AN EXISTENTIAL PSYCHOANALYTIC APPROACH

Actively Engaging and Supporting
Patients in Facing Their Mortality

The challenge for the psychoanalyst is to help the dying patient balance two mutually contradictory challenges: recognize that there is no cure for their illness and that life expectancy is short and "uncertain," and at the same time, make the best use of healthy time by concentrating on quality of life. This creative treatment both faces the fear of death directly and defends against it by shoring up the patient's "sense that, despite their physical maladies and limited life span, they are persons of value in a world of meaning with vital connections to friends and family" (Maxfied, Pyszczynski, & Solomon, in chapter 5 of this book). This view is espoused by the authors of the chapter on terror management and is in concert with my clinical experience.

I recommend that the psychoanalyst needs to consider focusing on the following details when treating a patient facing death: 1) engage the patient in facing their mortality (this includes an attempt to understand the patient's conception of death; is there an afterlife, continued suffering, isolation, suffering, reunion, heaven?), permit and encourage grieving while fostering the split or dissociation that preserves a part of the self (the mental self from the body self); 2) maintain a commonsense approach to denial that allows for fantasy formation, intermittent denial, and keeps the quality of life in the foreground; 3) actively collaborate with them in their search for meaning (a common and important natural desire for most patients at the end of life, it defends against death anxiety), and explore how they can try to transcend their illness; 4) engage them in their natural tendency to review their life experiences and accomplishments so that they can feel validated (help them to see that that they have left meaningful ripples or a legacy, so that there is something of them that continues on); and, finally, 5) ensure that a secure attachment or a regressive transference is encouraged as it buffers separation from loved ones in death and allows for a peaceful death.

FACING MORTALITY

When the patient is going through the transition from the expectation of cure to palliation, they can be expected to discuss their feelings of grief at having to accept that they will not return to their previous state of health. Grieving is necessary and should be encouraged. The patients may grieve about the loss of their health, their future, their important relationships, and the places they will miss or never see again, life goals that remain unfinished, and so forth. They may be bitter and angry. They may feel guilty about abandoning their families or unfinished business. These sessions provide an important emotional relief for the patient who cannot usually express these feelings toward important others as they are often in grief themselves and are usually unavailable for this type of discussion (Straker, 1998, 2008). They will also be facing the existential crisis that comes with the recognition that they are not going to be cured: the crisis of aloneness, the crisis that they will lose everyone and everything they care about, and the inevitability of death and questions of meaning.

At some point, grief will be interrupted by denial, disavowal, or dissociation. These defenses permit a split in the ego that permits a fantasy of immortality (Freud, 1915). This period allows the individual to mourn the dying body in favor of the newly created fantasy, which defends against death anxiety. At the same time, these defenses also allow for a very intense period of focus on living in the here-and-now, connecting with loved ones, and appreciating nature. A commonsense approach to denial, dissociation, and disavowal, especially if the patient is using it in the service of adaptive coping, is recommended. Interpretation of denial for the sake of truth, as in Minerbo's article, serves no good purpose, and it increases death anxiety when the patients are defending themselves (Straker & Wyszneski, 1986). Death anxiety can also be lessened by a positive transference with the analyst devoted to understanding and connected caring relationships with the medical staff, family, and friends.

Hagglund (1981) suggests that

> in order that the dying patient can mourn his ever-weakening, dying body, he must solve the narcissistic conflict between his weak and ailing body and the wished-for ideal state. He must create a fantasy of his own body as a cleansed or better form on some other level of existence or in a condition in which the body self-attains a specific libidinal value. Such a fantasy could be a religious rationalization . . . a fantasy of heaven, a return to a flawless nature. Another fantasy is of a mental self, of survival by means of creativity, through one's children, one's achievements, and the mental image imprinted in the minds of other people.

Some patients, paradoxically, seem to show a lessening of anxiety after they have come to accept that they are going to die. They describe a kind of psychological freedom that they never experienced before. They show a tendency to focus on the big picture; neurotic concerns of the past seem to be much less relevant. Many patients will speak about their greater appreciation of nature, family, and friends. Illness and death concerns create close intimate caring attachments with caretakers. Many dying patients become more spiritual and turn to God and religion. In fact, some have described the belief that they feel the presence of God. A video clip that illustrates this point is by William Webb, MD, a consultation, liaison psychiatrist in *On the Edge of Being: When Doctors Confront Cancer* (Straker & Drazen, 1991). In it he says, "I woke up today and felt a sense of calm. I felt God's presence; this is not some psychological reaction, this is real." Here we see the protective function of a belief in God. Such patients have accepted death with a fantasy that is protective. This kind of spirituality, a kind of connectedness to something greater than ourselves, can be seen to emerge in very sick people who are pinning for a "parent" (Fricchione, 2011). Some patient's talk about their readiness to die. Many, in fact, express the desire to die rather than persist in endless suffering.

It is of interest that the palliative care literature refers to the same processes as have been noted in my update. The descriptive terms are, of course, different, as each discipline has its own language. Bal Mount, the father of palliative care, talks about the goal of helping the patient die "healed." Healing is the product of caring—a caring that is spiritually inspired in the loving response of the caregiver (Peabody, 1927). Mount writes about broadening the approach of the physician from curing to resolving suffering. Patients who have terminal cancer suffer as long as they have not come to terms with the fact that they are dying. Up until that time, they have focused on an unachievable goal of cure and returning to earlier functioning, which they know is not going to happen. When they accept the fact that they are going to die, a new sense of integrity and wholeness emerges. That process involves a movement toward a life with a greater sense of connection and meaning, a new relationship to wounding, suffering, and an openness to the real hope possible in every moment (Mount, Hutchinson, & Kearney, 2011).

Several case vignettes that follow will illustrate how death anxiety and demoralization can be lessened by a split in the ego that permits this transitional illusion of survival of a part of the self. This is facilitated by a creative interaction with the analyst. The discussions convey a shared cultural heritage where the analyst validates a meaningful life that has been well-lived. This discussion increases self-esteem, helps define a legacy, encourages transcendence, and decreases death anxiety. This process is similar to what Solomon, Greenberg, and Pyszcynski (1998) have noted defends against death anxiety.

Case 1

Mr. X, a semi-retired internist and emeritus professor of medicine, was referred for psychotherapy after a diagnosis of a very aggressive cancer with six months to live. As a former analytic patient, he quickly became reinvested in the analysis. Picking up on the themes in his previous analysis, we were able to make the last six months of his life "the best he ever had" (his quote).

He was stoic, hardworking, and a very private person who tended to have difficulty with intimacy. He recalled his analyst urging him be more hedonistic and be open to greater intimacy. We began our work in the office three times a week. At that time, he was still trying to work while he was in great physical discomfort. Characteristically, he kept his illness a secret and he was reluctant to spend any money on himself, even at this time.

He had very good feelings about his first analysis and he credited it with helping him to have the wonderful career and family. He initially wanted to continue his office work for as long a time as he was able and not let his partners down. He acknowledged his prognosis on the one hand but denied the immediate need to take important life decisions on the other. As his advocate re quality of life (I took a commonsense approach), I confronted his denial as maladaptive. It failed to open up the possibilities of personal growth. I reminded him repeatedly that his limited healthy time might better be spent in what his former analyst might have termed hedonistic activities rather than work, especially while he still had some strength.

I encouraged him to consider taking his two children and grandchildren to the Caribbean in the midst of winter. This idea had initially seemed far too indulgent for him. He, however, did eventually agree to the trip, seeing it as a furthering of the psychoanalytic treatment goals and a pursuit of a better quality of life. He took his entire family, including grandchildren, to Jamaica. The trip proved to be a great success.

Upon returning to my office, we began to work through his issues about secrecy, stoicism, and intimacy. I actively engaged him in finding meaning in his last days, dealing with unfinished business, and saying goodbye to important relationships. I reminded him that it was not collegial to one day just drop out without saying anything. Secrecy was contrary to loyalty. He was obligated to reveal his condition to his colleagues. Similarly, this was also the only fair thing to do for his friends. He reluctantly agreed. Finally, with my prodding, he made it known to colleagues and friends that he was dying of cancer and that he would be interested in having visitors. A steady stream of friends, colleagues and partners, and former students began visiting his home. He was delighted by their expressions of love, friendship, and admiration. Never had he experienced the joy of this level of intimacy nor did he ever believe he was well liked. He felt very good about the life he had led and his legacy. As his condition progressed, he found it more and more difficult to visit my office and on one occasion had bowel incontinence in my office. Sessions continued on a daily basis at home.

As he became weaker, my daily visits at his home became briefer. He eagerly looked forward to continuing "the analysis," which he claimed was the most rewarding experience of his life (his quote). While he knew his prognosis, he never felt panicky about dying and was totally invested in the present, the visitors, and the analysis. He was so involved in living that he denied his imminent death. He had transcended his physical condition and enjoyed every moment. I chose to take a commonsense approach to his defense and not initiate a goodbye. One day I arrived for our usual meeting and I was told that he had died an hour earlier. We had not said our goodbyes because I presumed that, in his mind, the analysis would go on forever. One could say this man died healed.

This case demonstrates many of the principles I have included in my active creative approach with patients facing death. I did not hesitate to encourage the patient to face the issues that were still highly conflicted in his life in a psychoanalytic process. I interpreted his procrastination about spending money as a conflict about experiencing pleasure and a possible missed opportunity to be with his family for a warm winter vacation. I also addressed his conflicts with intimacy, privacy, and stoicism in relation to his upbringing and relationship with his father. This process allowed him to be free to enjoy his final weeks with colleagues, friends, and family. We also dealt with the end of his life with conversations that validated his life, allowed him to see his legacy, and, finally, be more intimate with students, colleagues, and family. As his health deteriorated, home visits became necessary. He often talked about continuing the analysis as if time would never stop. I saw no benefit in interfering with his fantasy and interpreting his denial. Daily visits, which he requested in lieu of hospice care, encouraged a regressive transference and a secure attachment. I believe that my relationship and the analysis helped him form a transitional fantasy of a never-ending relationship and analysis with his former analyst and me.

TRANSCENDING THE PRESENT
CIRCUMSTANCE WHEN POSSIBLE

Three other vignettes in addition to Mr. X's demonstrate how an analyst can attempt to help dying patients transcend their present intolerable life situation. Two of my dying patients were extremely troubled by their poor physical appearance and weakness. Each had separately stated on a number of occasions how they could barely recognize themselves when they saw their image in a mirror. I thought that by engaging them in frequent conversations about their past, particularly about the activities they were most proud, I could take them away from their present unacceptable situation even if only for the time of our session.

One of the patients had been an outstanding skier. The other man had been an extremely handsome man who prided himself on his seductiveness with women. When I met with the skier, I would often inquire about the races and runs he had skied. Being a skier myself, we often compared ski resorts and trails we both had skied. During those moments, he lived the memories of the past and felt as though he was the skier of old times. Similarly, the ladies' man was encouraged to retell his stories about his various love affairs and conquests. He liked nothing better than to recount those memories in detail. He too was reliving while retelling his experiences. These therapy experiences were a respite from the anguish and suffering and a refuge for him even when he was alone. Both men looked forward to my visits as an opportunity to transcend their unacceptable reality, if even for a short time.

In a somewhat similar manner, I helped several mothers who knew they were dying and were anguished about not being present at important events in their children's future. I recommended that they either videotape or write letters to their children to fit special occasions in the future. These interventions engaged them in overcoming their anguish and made the time left meaningful while, at the same time, gave the mothers some solace that they would be available to their offspring in the future (e.g., at bar mitzvahs, sweet sixteens, going to college, getting married, etc.). It gave this otherwise meaningless, anguished time a purpose and made the remaining time very meaningful.

Last, an update would not be complete without a few words about the use of psychotropic medications. I have found them to be an especially valuable tool in the relief of anxiety, depression, insomnia, and delirium and highly synergistic with the psychoanalytic psychotherapy.

REFERENCES

Becker, E. (1973). *Denial of death*. New York: Simon and Schuster.

Eissler, K. (1955). *The psychiatrist and the dying patient*. New York: International University Press.

Freud, S. (1915). *Thoughts for our times, 14*. London: Hogarth Press, 299.

Fricchione, G. (2011). Separation attachment theory in illness and the role of the healthcare practitioner. In T. A. Hutchison (Ed.), *Whole person care: A new paradigm for the 21st century*. Quebec: Springer.

Gould, S. J. (1986). The medium isn't the message. *Discover, 6*.

Hagglund, T. B. (1981). The final stages of the dying process. *International Journal of Psychoanlaysis, 62*, 45.

Hutchinson, T. A., Mount, B. M., & Kearney, M. (2011). The healing journey. In T. A. Hutchinson (Ed.), *Whole person care: A new paradigm for the 21st century*. Quebec: Springer.

Keating, N., Landrum, M. B., Rogers, S. O., Jr., Baum, S. K., Virnig, B. A., Huskamp, H. A., et al. (2010). Physicians factors associated with discussions about the end of life care. *Cancer, 1*.

Massie, M. J., Holland, I. C., & Straker, N. (1989). Psychotherapeutic intervention. In J. C. Holland & J. R. Rowland (Eds.), *Handbook on Psycho--Oncology*. New York: Oxford University Press.

Mayer, E. L. (1994). Some implications for psychoanalytic technique drawn from analysis of a dying patient. *Psychoanalytic Quarterly, 63*, 1.

Minerbo, V. (1998). The patient without a couch: An analysis of a patient with terminal cancer.*international Journal of Psychoanalysis, 79*, 83–89.

Norton, J. (1963). The treatment of a dying patient. *Psychoanalytic Study of the Child, 18*, 541.

Peabody, F. W. (1927). The care of the patient. *Journal of the American Medical Association, 88*, 877–882.

Roose, L. (1969). The dying patient. *International Journal of Psychoanalysis, 50*(3), 385–397.

Solomon, S., Greenberg, J., & Pyszcynski, T. (1998). Tales from the crypt: On the role of death in life. *Zygon, 33*, 1.

Straker, N. (1990). *On the edge of being when doctors confront cancer.* Video presentation.

———. (1998). Psycho-dynamic psychotherapy for cancer patients. *Journal of Psychotherapy Practice and Research, 7*, 11–9.

———. (2005). *The courage to survive: Facing the death of your soul mate.* Video website (www.international psychoalysis.net).

———. (2008). Dynamic psychodynamic for cancer patients and their partners. *Psychiatric Times, 8*(9), 14–18.

———. (2011). The courage to survive: Facing the loss of your soul mate. *Palliative and Supportive Care, 9*(2): 119–121.

Straker, N., & Drazen, R. (1991). On the edge of being: When doctors confront cancer. Video.

Straker, N., & Wysznski, A. (1986). A denial in the cancer patient: A commonsense approach. *International Medicine for the Specialist, 7*, 150–155.

III

Case Presentations Section

Chapter Eight

"... That Darkness Is About to Pass" [1]

The Treatment of a Dying Patient

Abby Adams-Silvan, PhD

This chapter describes the psychoanalytic psychotherapy of a middle-age woman ill with cancer. The patient entered treatment frightened, depressed, and feeling unable to endure the narcissistic humiliation of chemotherapy. She actively wished to abandon the struggle for life in spite of the real possibility of a significant remission. Passive longings dominated her thoughts, but a good family situation mobilized a wish to continue the struggle. It was the immediate goal of the treatment to strengthen that wish by mobilizing healthy narcissistic cathexes that would facilitate feelings of self-esteem, personal pride, and pleasure in living. The treatment was conducted on a twice-weekly basis for almost three years. After two years, it was determined that the illness was terminal, and the patient expressed the wish to be helped to "let go," precisely the reverse of the goal toward which we had previously been working. This chapter describes the processes by which the patient was able to use the two stages of her treatment to accomplish her goals: to feel greater pride in life and then, with the help of a physician, to die as she had wished. Her final messages reflected her feeling that her suicide was a loving and estimable act.

> Presentiment—is that long Shadow—on the Lawn—
> Indicative that Suns go down—
> The Notice to the startled Grass
> That Darkness—is about to pass—
> —Emily Dickinson

When I first saw Mrs. M., she was sitting alone in my waiting room, wrapped in a voluminous, richly colored fur coat which she held about herself blanket-like, as though she were chilled. She was a pale, well-groomed, slender, very attractive middle-age woman with auburn hair which was not easily identifiable as the wig I knew it must be.

Her face was a mask of boredom, but when she became aware of my presence, her expression changed. She smiled engagingly, held out her hand and introduced herself, murmured a socially appropriate greeting, and walked with me down the hall to my office as though to the best table for a cheerful lunch and gossip.

When I invited her to speak about herself, Mrs. M. told me that it would be more helpful if I asked her questions since she did not know what I needed to hear. I explained that it would be more useful if she would simply tell me about herself as it spontaneously occurred to her. She shrugged and began by saying, "I am a butterfly. I am useless," and she repeated, "A butterfly."

Mrs. M. went on to say that there was very little she could think to tell me: she had no vocational or avocational interests that she felt were of significance. She gave successful parties, of which she was quite proud, and went to parties, which she enjoyed, and she traveled a good deal, with much pleasure. She was, however, too ill now from her chemotherapy to enjoy or participate in any of that, and it was a great loss. She had always devoted herself to her home and her husband, child, and friends. She had one daughter; early in her marriage she had suffered three late miscarriages.

Mrs. M. was now forty-nine years old, and in the preceding months she had had surgery for a kidney cancer. She was in the midst of a course of chemotherapy that left her weak, ill, "and ugly, so ugly. Just look at this wig—my hair used to be so beautiful when I was little." She was hopeful, but doubtful, that the "second look" surgery would show remission. The cancer had been silent for quite a while before it was dramatically discovered. She had, of course, been frightened and depressed for some time, but she had had no intention of seeking psychotherapeutic help until a particular incident precipitated a keenly felt need for "something—someone to talk to—something."

In the incident she reported, she had been taking a walk with her husband and had seen in a store window a suit she found very much to her taste. They went into the store to make inquiries. She told me the price of the suit, several thousand dollars, in a completely bland way; her husband had urged her to buy it, but instead of proceeding to do so, as she said she would ordinarily have done, she suddenly thought, "But where will I wear it? I can't go out, I can't count on feeling well enough." She turned abruptly and left the store. That evening she called a friend (who was not a mental health professional) to ask if she knew someone who would "be willing to see me." The incident symbolized for her a potent deprivation of major significance. More important, I think, it signaled the mobilization of a conflict around her wish to remain withdrawn, hidden, and protected from the world, and a weaker but significant contradictory wish to reengage and fight for her life.

During that first interview she told me that she had never before thought to seek psychotherapeutic help. Her life was, she said, "perfect." She had "married late" for those days—that is, at thirty. Before marrying she had lived with her widowed mother, commuting to a small girls' college where she had studied to become an early childhood educator in case she needed to support herself, and then worked only until she married. She much disliked the work, and her husband encouraged her to depend on him, as she gratefully did.

Until Mrs. M. married, she had never felt that she could safely be dependent, but after her marriage she had consciously been very happy to relinquish her worries and struggles around trying to be independent to rely on her husband. Her relationship with her mother, who died just several years before her own illness was discovered, had been intense, stormy, and, as far as she was aware, almost totally negative. She had, however, lived with her, "because Mother wished it." She did not realize, when we first spoke, how bound she actually was to her mother, whom she described as controlling, harsh, critical, negative, and "mean." At that first interview she told me an anecdote involving coming home from school to "that dark, bleak house" because she was sick. She only wanted her mother to care for her and waited in the dim hall on a chair for hours until her mother came home. Immediately after telling me this memory, she looked around my office and told me how her mood was very much influenced by her surroundings and how much she liked the decor of my office. She found the colors attractive and bright but soothing, and she smiled for the first time during the interview.

Mrs. M. told me that she hardly remembered her father at all, though he had lived until her twenties. She had one or two memories, but he was "nothing—a blank—just not important to me." Then, in immediate sequence, surely with transference implications, Mrs. M. asked me how I could possibly help her. She had talked so much, she said, but what could I do for her?

I explained that I would try to understand and would never underestimate the reality of her situation. It was hard, painful, frightening, and realistically miserable. I assured her that I would never forget that she carried these real and heavy burdens. However, I went on, I might be able to help in two ways. First, having someone to speak to in any way she chose, without reference to my feelings, could allow her to put into words feelings and ideas that she wanted and needed to express but might find difficult or impossible with someone toward whom she felt she should be protective. There might be some thoughts that she would find unacceptable to express to people with whom she had mutually loving and protective relationships—her daughter, husband, friends—whereas she would not have to fear hurting or frightening me. I added that she would probably not be able to believe that, but she should hear me say it. In fact, if she should find herself restricting what she said or how she said it, that would be important for us to know, because it would aid us in the second and very important way I thought I might be able to offer her help.

This second way was that, in addition to all the real misery she was enduring, she probably was carrying some unnecessary burdens from the past, burdens that might be further draining her strength. If she decided to work with me, we might be able to ease some old emotional pressures and leave her freer to engage in her present battles. For instance, although I respected her feelings to the contrary, in my judgment she looked very attractive. There must be reasons beyond reality, things in her past, that made her feel so ugly. I reassured her that I was not trying to convince her of something she did not feel; rather, I wanted to call her attention to a strong feeling that was important to her, a painful burden, and—to my eyes—unnecessary for her to bear.

Her response to my first statement was dismissive: she did not think she could speak to a stranger without being reasonably polite and taking the feelings of the other into consideration. On the other hand, she found it interesting to think about the other way I could help. In a cool but involved tone, she told me how important it was to her to feel beautiful and how ugly she had felt as a child—"only my hair was good." She "confessed" that she had been shy and "clumsy" and that she had had what she perceived as a large unsightly mole on her face, which had not been removed until adolescence. Her mother had been unsympathetic, telling the little girl it didn't matter until later, when it would be "taken care of." Could that, Mrs. M. wondered, be the sort of thing I meant? Indeed it was, I assured her. Feelings about the ugly growth of her childhood might somehow be influencing her current perception of herself. She was intrigued but very calm. We had made a connection, however, and I expressed excitement about the immediate relevance of this historical material, an excitement that I hoped would engage her. I found out later that, in fact, it did, but she could not show it openly at the time.

Still apparently detached, she said she thought she would like to see me regularly, but that there would be times when she would be just too weak to come. I told her I would come to her home or to the hospital if she wanted me to; we could simply decide as circumstances and her wishes dictated. We settled on two visits a week. "But you will see, I may not be interesting enough for that," she warned me in a flat and factual way, neither humorous nor apologetic.

What emerged very vividly in the second session was how much she wanted to give up her fight against her cancer, a giving-up that at that time was premature. She accepted that treatment might still effect a significant remission; her family was ardently trying to keep her fighting, but she did so, she said, only for them. She herself was tired, discouraged, weak, horribly bored, and cut off from her previous sources of pleasure and—I added—of self-worth. She expressed surprise at this, but agreed. Although she had never felt useful, she hadn't cared; she enjoyed her life very much. Now, she said, she just had nothing to feel proud of.

I began to speak about pride, asking her to tell me what she had felt proud of in her life. She shrugged, palms up, elbows tight to her body, smiled in a contemptuous-appearing way, and seemed, by that gesture, to challenge me to find something she was really proud of. She thought she might be a good wife and mother, but . . . I remarked that it must be very hard to fight for your life when you feel your life is so inestimable. Yes, she agreed. Well, I went on, this must go far back, and we must explore it; there were things to understand. Meanwhile, she should know that, if nothing else, the fact that every waking moment was so hard meant to me that she was calling on considerable courage that came from somewhere. This is an example of how I regularly invited analysis in conjunction with a statement of support.

Mrs. M. said that the word "courage" was totally wrong. Then, in an uncharacteristically animated way, she leaned forward and said that she was going to tell me something personal. She could not remember a day in her life when she had not been frightened. Not all day, but every day she experienced a miserable sense of fear for some length of time. So, she told me, I could see that she was far from courageous. I told her that to me it seemed quite the opposite: to face every day with some measure of anxiety took a fair amount of courage. She had a right to know I felt that way, but I was not, I told her again, trying to convince her. I said I knew that was impossible and that only with exploration and understanding might her feelings change. This again, I said, was an example of the extra burdens we had discussed. She had a past, a complex history, and there were answers to seek within herself.

It is obvious that I was, at this time, taking a very active stance in the treatment and was finding as many opportunities as possible to make positive comments to the patient about herself, trying thereby to serve as a supportive positive transference figure and a benign auxiliary ego/superego. I was taking care to remain in the repeated context of historical dynamics while trying to draw her into self-examination. Since the patient was certainly critically ill and perhaps dying, an attempt to move beyond supportive, primarily abreactive techniques might be questionable. My therapeutic goal at this time was to mobilize a healthy narcissistic investment so that Mrs. M. could experience some sense of energetic participation in her cancer treatment and could fight harder to live. That her attitude at this point was bitterly acquiescent to her illness presented a real problem.

It was my conviction that this goal of maximizing positive, healthy narcissistic cathexes would be well served if I could truly interest her in herself, in her intrapsychic processes, and object relations. If she could feel that she was self-lovable and become excited about herself, then she could fight harder. I understood that this goal might have to be reversed, that if her illness took a negative course I would be in the position of having to help her let go of life after a time when I had been trying to help her hold tight. She had, indeed, expressed the intention to commit suicide if the disease went too far and had undertaken to provide herself with the means to do so. I felt I must quickly and actively reach out to engage her in a therapeutic process.

Starting in her second session, she complained about the care she was receiving from the hospital, physicians, and nurses. She experienced them all as brusque, uninterested, and harsh. The transference implications were clear; negative feelings about me would be easily aroused into conscious awareness and, I believed, must be warded off if possible, since she could readily bolt from treatment. She had made it clear that she had little capacity to tolerate interpersonal discomfort.

Given the nature of what seemed to be a narcissistic/hysterical character structure, I decided that it was very important to continue to mobilize positive transference. On the other hand, I did not want to reinforce perceptions that were making her life harder by evoking the very harshness about which she complained. I expressed sympathy with her experiences as she reported them, emphasizing in my choice of words that this was her inner experience, that I accepted that experience as real, and that, unpleasant though it was, perhaps here again was an extra burden. Perhaps, for instance, she had had harsh experiences with other caretakers in her past and had been drained of the energy to tolerate necessary but unpleasant treatment, her store of patience depleted by remembered and unremembered experiences. I stressed that unpleasant expectations based on the past could be making the present even harder.

Here again it will be noted that I was moving quickly to explore her transferential displacement onto new authority figures other than myself at the same time that I expressed sympathy and suggested unknown reasons for her despair.

Indeed, Mrs. M. began to speak of her mother and how angry and harsh she had been. In fact, she told me, she had been that way with everyone in the family: my patient, her older brother, her mother's brother, even, eventually, her friends. She quarreled with everyone.

The only person her mother treated well was Mrs. M.'s father, whom she "worshiped and adored." "Him," she said, "she kept for herself. He was handsome, very handsome." As it turned out, I was to hear about the intensely angry character of Mrs. M.'s mother many times and strikingly little about her father.

What I began to glean of my patient's character was an identification built on frustrated and frightened longing for closeness to her critical, angry mother and to the father who she felt had been clearly declared off-limits. His absence from her conscious memory symbolized her conflicted acceptance of his forbidden status, as well as other meanings. Her apparent bouts of anxiety signaled the degree to which her conflicts were active.

Her controlled appearance was antithetical to the behavior she reported. Mrs. M. told me she had a "terrible temper" and easily became enraged. I, however, saw only the reflection of this rage and defenses against its expression. One day, for example, the air-conditioning in my waiting room was set too low, and Mrs. M. said she had gotten a chill waiting for me. She was obviously very, very angry. This seemed an overreaction to what was nevertheless a real experience of my causing her physical discomfort, and I thought it worthwhile to encourage her expression of her feeling, noting that she indeed looked very angry and very cold. She simply agreed, tight-lipped, turned her head away, and said she had nothing to talk about. When I pushed a bit to try to help her to speak of her discomfort, she said in a withering way that "it is hardly so important as all that," thereby expressing contempt, protection of me, the rendering of me impotent, and the deprivation of herself, all in eight words.

I tried to engage her by noting that this was analogous to the other physical treatment she was receiving and that it might be useful to examine it from this point of view, but she simply could not do so. It was not the same; she never doubted my good intent, and she knew (correctly enough) that I would change the setting on the air conditioner since she had mentioned it. I noted that she might have responded differently in other situations, but she only shrugged. Her tendency to split the good and bad objects had by then been amply indicated, and here it was before us, but proving unusable. With me she maintained stringent self-control, but one could see—in this as in other situations—how that self-control was also in the service of controlling others. All in all, the incident enacted a good deal.

This incident also illustrates a very real technical problem, since I had virtually arranged the therapeutic situation in a way that could readily make the important expression of a negative feeling difficult. I had tried hard, by my tone, to indicate my acceptance of her negative feelings, but that itself could mitigate them too much. It remains a technical dilemma. My patient had a history of terminating unsatisfactory relationships abruptly (though she could also be deeply loyal) and had a real need for a positive therapeutic relationship, but at the same time was fearful of closeness, holding herself aloof, even pushing away, especially in a competitive situation. (She had remarked occasionally that she supposed I saw many people, and, although highly conflicted, she was competitive with others and, I assumed, with me.) I had deliberately actively tried to engage her positive feelings, but in so doing I had made it extremely difficult to analyze a crucial hostile aspect of her character. How to negotiate this Scylla and Charybdis, which has threatened to wreck many a psychoanalytic voyager, is surely a matter for discussion and careful thought.

On the positive side, I was sometimes quite successful in helping Mrs. M. to face the physical unpleasantness of her medical treatment in spite of her continuing reports of interpersonal problems with the professionals involved. As we explored the deeper meaning of her experiences, she gained the stamina to tolerate the genuinely distressing procedures and seemed to revive—in the literal sense of the word—her will to live.

One example of how we worked is particularly vivid. Mrs. M. was about to undergo a second series of chemotherapy treatments. She expressed the feeling that she just couldn't take it, and I asked her to describe to me exactly what was going to happen and what the procedure was going to entail as she remembered it. I had learned by then that if I started by asking her to describe what she imagined or tried to force a fantasy, I would get only a shrug; she was simply too fearful of her spontaneous fantasy life and correspondingly inhibited in it to use it without my active help.

In any case, I asked her to take me step-by-step through the procedure. Halting often, she described how she would sign into the hospital, have to get into bed, how the nurse would insert the needle . . . (pause) "And then?" (pause) "I just lie there." (pause) "And then?" "Nothing, the needle is in." (pause) "Please tell me—what next?" "Well, the needle—nothing—it just starts . . . "

At this point I myself had a vivid fantasy image of her lying rigid, stock-still, self-immobilized to an unnecessary degree. I suspect that I had constructed this image from her tone, her body tension, and her characteristic (but therefore even more meaningful) lack of spontaneity. It was as though she was demonstrating for me a kind of lifelessness. I mentioned that she seemed to be immobilized just in telling me; how, in fact, did she lie on the bed? She said that actually she was quite "stiff" during the treatment; it was very hard for her to relax. Again she stopped. I told her I had noticed she mentioned the needle several times. Was there, I wondered, something special about that? To my surprise she laughed (an event that occurred very, very seldomly) and said that while I was talking she had the oddest thought. Again she stopped. What? Well, she had thought of Frankenstein, lying on the operating table, not yet alive, with all the needles in him. She had, of course, confused the doctor with the monster, and added the needles and operating table. Her identification with the monster was apparent, although I hoped that this was indicative of an identification with the life-giving doctor as well. She shuddered when she thought of the monster and how he was never really alive. Stop again. And then? In the end, she recalled, he had killed a little girl, she thought by accident, and he had to be burned. Again she shuddered. I could not help, of course, thinking of her own early sadness as a little girl and of her later miscarriages.

I told her it seemed to me that some things about all that connected with the intensity of her difficulty with her treatments; did she have any thoughts about that? No, but it made sense. Again, dead stop. It was, I said, as though there was some connection to her own feeling of being "monstrous." I chose that element because of her emphasis on ugliness and scarring, her equation of stupidity, helplessness, and destruction connected with affection (the murder of the child), being "stuck" between life and death, and her sense of not being able to live now even though she was alive. All this indicated her identification with the helpless but monstrous creature. Indeed, with a little help, she was finally able to speak quite movingly about just those issues. Later she reported that the chemotherapy treatment had indeed been not as bad as usual.

Our work continued. It was consistently necessary for me to be quite active since she was dominated by the need to maintain a passive-receptive attitude, an attitude that did not bode well in her fight against illness. On the other hand, she no longer spoke of abandoning her cancer treatment, and although she continued to experience the practitioners she had to deal with as detached, unsympathetic, and not interested in her, her tolerance for this increased.

Gradually, new dimensions of her history emerged on which I could focus in the service of my stated goal: to intensify healthy narcissistic cathexes. I approached this by returning again and again to the issue of pride when I felt the manifest content of the session warranted it.

On one occasion we were speaking yet again of her feelings of uselessness, and I remarked once more on how good it was that we could continue to explore the reasons that she did not feel she deserved to live. This time she remarked dryly that she was simply not desirable now, and she had proof: she was losing her friends. They did not seem to understand that she could not entertain as before or that she would frequently have to break lunch dates. She claimed that they had stopped making appointments because she canceled too often at the last minute because of weakness. I observed that she seemed to feel that this behavior was understandable. She agreed; why, of course it was understandable. They didn't like to be with her, though she tried to be interesting and "amusing," and her illness made her socially unreliable. Why should they wish to see her? Did I not understand that? It will be recalled that her concern with being interesting and reliable with me had been expressed at our first consultation. Somewhere, she was afraid that I, too, would reject her.

I remarked on her conviction that sickness was intolerable to others, thinking to move to the externalization I thought was involved. What emerged, however, was that her father—though not her mother—had been a Christian Scientist, that she had regularly attended Christian Science Sunday school for many years of her childhood, and that only there did she remember having friendships, and feeling liked. At that time, she said, she certainly believed the theology she was taught, though "of course, as an adult I know better." Although she did not really remember, she believed her father always took her. She thought, in retrospect, that he did not accept the doctrine and had joined the church "for business reasons," but he did attend services regularly. It emerged more directly that "business reasons" had to do with anti-Semitism and that her father had felt it necessary to hide the fact that he was Jewish.

In other words, it was probable that her illness provoked guilt that had oedipal implications, as well as more readily available reasons for self-condemnation and the most obvious reason for shame: illness is badness. Sickness displays for all to see that one is spiritually inadequate, and being Jewish is another danger.

Here again, I was faced with a technical choice: I could focus on her relationship to her father; I could attempt to sort out the interpersonal reality—was it her friends who stopped calling or she?—and utilize the transference implications; I could work with her obviously conflicted exhibitionism; or I could deal with her shame as related to her early religious beliefs and move to other sources of shame and their connection to her present situation. Because of the passive attitude I have described, and because she warded off her own capacity for insightful reflection, the choice of topic, as so often happened, was mine.

Clinically, I now believe that this is a technical situation that may characterize the psychotherapeutic treatment of a seriously—perhaps terminally—ill patient. There is a time pressure that may indicate, or even mandate, the relative abandonment of the attitude of neutrality, at least with respect to subject matter. In this situation equidistance from id, ego, and superego feels impossible and unwarranted. For my patient at that time, I was certainly emphasizing superego issues, with the goal of allowing id material to emerge so as to maximize her capacity for pride and pleasure experiences and thereby keep her engaged with life. One way or another, right or wrong, I felt myself to be in the position where I simply had to continue to accept the active role she wished me to take, although I surely recognized it as a transference recreation probably related to exhibitionistic/voyeuristic conflicts.

In this respect, the technical decisions required in such treatment resemble those that are generally made with patients whose pathology is dynamically related to more preoedipal issues than I believed to be the case with Mrs. M. Perhaps we might even speculate that severe and/or terminal illness regularly reinforces and exacerbates preoedipal issues in all patients—in other words, that the manifest psychological regression of the physically ill person reflects a real change in psychic structure that has rearranged the alignments in the mind, possibly bringing to the fore the earliest object imagoes and subsequent identifications. If so, caretaking will be seen as poor

if the early caretakers were inadequate. This situation will then be reproduced internally in the patient's care of herself and externally in a compulsive repetition in relationships to current caretakers, both of which were true
of Mrs. M. vis-à-vis her illness.

I was aware that I myself felt a kind of relaxation from a long personal
and professional accumulation of technical guidelines, experience, requirements, and even strictures. I was also aware, however, that I had to be
especially alert to my own complementary and/or countertransference responses, which I found to be stimulated a great deal more than under more
usual treatment circumstances. Perhaps I felt in this treatment as the earliest
analysts did: my own experience was limited; I had a global map but little
except a few classic psychoanalytically oriented descriptions to mark specific
routes (Brodsky, 1959; Eissler, 1955; Norton, 1968; Roose, 1969; Sandford,
1957). Only my patient could guide me. Like all who strike out in relatively
uncharted psychological territory, I knew that she would instruct me if I
would only listen, but I had to be prepared to not always understand her
directions. As Bach (1985) says, "My primary debt is to my patients who,
with extraordinary courage and forbearance, have persevered in teaching me
how to analyze them" (p. xix).

In any case, with regard to her memories of her father and her experience
with Christian Science, I chose to explore Mrs. M.'s sense of guilt about
being sick, with reference to childhood and adolescent religious beliefs. I
thought this would be most readily available and acceptable to her to work
with. We even were able to discuss the sickness incident she mentioned at
our first consultation, she again was able to make a new connection, and she
reported subsequently that she experienced a palpable sense of relief. Once
again, she found facing a new round of chemotherapy a little easier.

In retrospect, however, I believe that I did not stress sufficiently that
aspect of her interpersonal problems that was the result of the projection of
her conflicts, especially her sadomasochistic impulses. We did speak of her
infantile conviction that she would and should be punished for her sickness/
badness so that unconsciously she might find harsh treatment expectable and
justified, but we were never able to relate this to her subsequent rejection of
special help in any way that might enable her to change her behavior. That is,
her masochistic wish to evoke such treatment was not reachable.

She seemed to long for the active, loving mother and father who would
fight for her but compulsively repeated the absence of those figures. I believe
that given more time, she might have been able to examine more productively her own role in her caretaking problems, but it would have required much
help to get in touch with her desire/need for the unpleasant state, and a much
sturdier capacity than she had at that time to sustain narcissistic pain.

Meanwhile, her poor care of herself reflected an identification with a
malignant imago that I was trying hard to obscure at least somewhat by the

overlay of a new object representation in her experience and fantasy of me and of her husband as benign caretakers. I tried to do this by accepting whatever she told me of her "badness" and consistently voicing my concern for her ease and comfort and my confidence in her desirability and intellect, which I genuinely felt. (Eissler [1955] stresses how important it is not to be dishonest with a dying patient, as indeed it is with any patient, and I was careful always to observe this rule.) I generally indicated such positive feelings at moments when she had delightedly or quickly understood an interaction between us, especially if this involved noticing something not so positive about me.

Looking back, I regret my decision not to introduce in this context the subject of her miscarriages and her perception of her body as producing "ugly" moles and cancers instead of babies. At the time I felt that, in the absence of her spontaneously broaching the subject, I would undo an important suppression. I may, however, have missed an opportunity to explore further her sense of "uselessness" and to facilitate the potential sublimation of her frustrated maternal impulses.

During this time I visited her twice at her home, her chemotherapy having left her too weak to come to my office for appointments. She elected on those occasions to see me in a den that, in fact, was more like an alcove in that it was without doors. My outstanding memory of this den, other than its openness, was that there was a photograph of Mrs. M.'s mother displayed prominently. Beneath this picture was a cabinet where, Mrs. M. told me, she kept the pills she had obtained with which to kill herself. She was quite undramatic about this announcement, mentioning only that she hoped she would have the courage to take them before it was too late. She was terrified that she would die an "ugly, undignified, painful" death, as her mother had. I was aware at that time of the strong possibility that reunion fantasies were influencing Mrs. M.

At that session she told me that after her first surgery, while still in the hospital, she had had a very strong visual image of her mother at the door of her room. She went on to say that her second-look operation had been scheduled, and for the first time she felt really hopeful. She was, however, superstitious about saying that. Her mother had been superstitious, and she wanted me to know that she was, too. She was afraid to be hopeful.

I thought that all this articulated, behaviorally and verbally, her conflicts around exhibitionism and life-and-death fears and wishes. In addition, it suggested a strong transference experience and an attempt to internalize her fantasy of me, as I had hoped, in the struggle against her longing for and identification with her mother. This last was, in my opinion, particularly dangerous to her at this time because of her reunion fantasies.

Mrs. M.'s second-look surgery took place shortly after this session. Though we did not know it then, our work had crossed an invisible but ineradicable line.

Two days after her surgery I received a call from a member of Mrs. M.'s family. Mrs. M. was desperately upset, speaking of suicide. She did not want me to visit, a wish I honored but, in retrospect, do not think I should have. She had been told that the cancer was much attenuated but not as remitted as had been hoped. She would have to submit to additional—and more experimental—treatment. Her family and physicians, I was told, felt this was worth trying. She herself only wanted to die.

The family member I spoke with asked if antidepressant medication might help. I felt a consultation was indicated and arranged for her to see Dr. X., a medical analyst with a subspecialty in psychopharmacology for cancer patients. He prescribed an antidepressant, arranged a regime of follow-up appointments, and, most significantly offered help in negotiating the complexities of patient-physician, patient-hospital, and patient-"professional cancer community" relationships.

Mrs. M. was willing to try but was not sanguine. With the dashing of her hard-won hopes, she again reported in her sessions how she was receiving unsympathetic and unpleasant care. Though her husband and I remained on the positive valence of her split, all physicians and even hospital personnel were again experienced as negative. As a result of our work, her therapeutic time had come to be characterized less and less by complaints in that arena of her life. Now, when she needed practical help most, she was again rejecting those who offered it. This was particularly sad because she would now be under the care of a new physician who was indeed research-oriented, and it was necessary for her to change hospitals because of the experimental nature of her treatment.

Mrs. M. kept her appointments with me regularly, but now she spoke of feeling that she would die and of her need to believe that I would help her be decisive when she must finally take her pills and would staunchly ally myself with her determination to avoid a final agony. Over and over she spoke of her horror of the pain and physical deterioration of the last stages of cancer. She reported that her family supported her plan to kill herself should her condition worsen substantially, but that everyone but she was convinced that she should still fight, that there was hope. I was reliably informed that she still might be able to experience several years of comfortable remission, so I shared the family attitude as she described it.

I told Mrs. M. that I would do my best to help her "let go" when it seemed that all hope really was lost but that I was not convinced that the time had come. I had deep concerns that she would experience this as tremendously unempathic and that I would lose her trust. To my relief, she simply gestured her acquiescence, saying that I sounded like her family. She didn't agree, but . . . she was willing to go on a little longer.

At this time, Mrs. M. looked and felt fairly well. She was not suffering from the hair loss that so distressed her, and she was not bloated or nauseated, so her external appearance was objectively more than satisfactory and subjectively much more acceptable. Nevertheless, the treatments had left her with hidden but unpleasant side effects, such as mouth sores. When she told me about them, I asked what palliative care and symptomatic relief she was seeking, and she said nothing would help.

She was apparently becoming more and more passive in seeking what relief might be available. I again tried to help her to see that she was harshly mistreating herself as she had described her mother doing and was leaving potential caretakers out of her life, having in mind the compartmentalization of mother and father.

I was wrong, Mrs. M. said, about her not accepting care: her husband, her daughter, her closest friend, and I were of great help. But Drs. X., L., N., and P. and all the other medical personnel "were abrupt and self-interested." She did not wish to remain on antidepressants; she felt they "detached" her from herself. She did not want to be in contact with Dr. X., nor did she wish me to continue to communicate with him. I asked permission to speak with Dr. X. to tell him this. It was granted, and he expressed his deep regrets. Mrs. M. terminated that relationship and abandoned her psychotropic medication.

Her mood varied, but she never wept. She spoke more and more of the past, but not regretfully. There were many spontaneous negations: I'm not sorry I didn't become professional or have some kind of volunteer work; I'm not unhappy about living with my mother so long; I don't think I wasted my time; I've had a completely wonderful life. I felt that to analyze her defenses at this time was contraindicated. On the other hand, as always, defense signals conflict, and the unacceptable side of it may be threatening to erupt. She was certainly not so sure as all that.

She still required very active participation from me, and this closely reflected her character. She had not been an active participant in life; she had been too conflicted and anxious to invest libidinal energy in any extradomiciliary cause or interest. Because of the threat of eruption of despair over her sense of uselessness, I felt under some pressure to provide overt comfort, and I thought it might be helpful to ask whether she felt she had given pleasure and why she tended to feel that that was a useless attribute. This led fairly readily to her feeling that she could never really please her mother and that her father "didn't seem to care much to be with me, except—wait. . . ." She suddenly, abruptly remembered regularly meeting him at his office and riding home with him in her early teens. Other memories followed, and she eventually came to see both parents' attitude toward her as having more to do with their own inner struggles than with her acceptability. On one occasion she flashed a brilliant smile at me and said, "If I live, perhaps you can find me my father." That, and the moment when she said perhaps I might take a course in career counseling and advise her because she thought she might be potentially vocationally useful after all, were heady but bittersweet draughts during this phase. I always responded with a positive answer that echoed her own contingent "if I live . . .": "If you live, we'll go looking together . . ."

During this period, I had occasion to see her in the hospital sometimes when she had her treatments, which required several days' stay, and also at home. When she was particularly weak, I attended her in her bedroom. The multitude of symbolic meanings of all this was not discussed, but she told me she was glad I had seen her bedroom—it was the place she felt safest in the world. The first time I entered the room I was flabbergasted: though she had never mentioned it (significant in itself), the major color was the dominant one in my office. I had been very lucky indeed. Her original trust was based in part on a fortuitous coincidence that allowed a narcissistic identification to occur, and she was as safe with me as she would be alone. In fact, one might speculate that in some ways, she was alone.

Her CA-125 (cancer antigen-125) count did not go down after treatments with the experimental drug. This medication was extremely rare, and she was finally told she could have no more. "It would be wasted on me. I am dying." Then she said she knew I had not meant for her to find her father that way, but maybe she would. At that moment, I, too, gave up hope. What was emerging for Mrs. M. was reunion as a natural defense, what Roose (1969) speaks of as "the phenomena of regression and reunion in . . . dying patients" (p. 392). This is regularly reported in the literature (Brodsky, 1959; Gediman, 1981; Jones, 1911; Pollack, 1974, 1975; Sandford, 1957; Wald, 1957). Her unconscious longing to join her mother and father may have been a very strong dynamic in the way her entire illness had affected her, and when remission was a possibility, reunion as a wish had been dangerous. Now, as a protective device, it was easing her pain. This impulse toward reunion may, in fact, be a frequent dynamic in many very seriously ill patients, and that possibility should be regularly considered in psychotherapeutic treatment.

Mrs. M. went on, at that session, to acknowledge the relationships that now must be relinquished. She wanted to discuss planning for her husband and daughter, a task upon which she would concentrate, so that she could ease their way.

Mrs. M. consulted a sympathetic physician who advised her on her suicide: how to take her pills, how someone might have to help, and so on. It was particularly important to her that he told her he would sign the death certificate and that there would be no autopsy. She never asked my opinion or told me his name. She either assumed my empathy or had no interest in it. (I suspect a little of both.) I felt it was most important for her to feel that I did understand, or at least was trying hard to do so, but how? Her main request of me at this point was that I help her to feel strong enough to end her life before she became unable to do so. I was reliably informed that her disease was terminal, that there was no way to have a truly dependable timetable, but that she had, in all probability, less than a year to live; and that that year would be one of painful and acute deterioration. It was just this turn of events I'd been concerned about since I was neither experientially nor characterologically prepared for it. As had happened so frequently, my patient told me what to do for her.

She began to speak in her sessions about the death of a good friend the previous year from cancer, of how her friend had ended "a brilliant life" "writhing in agony," "calling for her mother," "ugly," "wasted," "out of touch with everyone around her," and "so alone, alone." She said that it was unbearable to picture herself in such a situation, and that to put her family through such scenes was "unconscionable." Juxtaposed with tormented images, she spoke of how best she might plan to ease the experience of her death for those she had depended on, loved, and to whom she felt close. She spoke of letters she would write, making it clear to friends and family that she hoped her husband would eventually marry again, and generally adopted a conscious attitude of altruism. She focused on her plans with a kind of satisfaction. She was doing what she had done for many years: planning an event that should go smoothly and even beautifully, at the same time protecting those she loved so that she could feel proud.

I had to consistently restrain myself from hindering a process that was, in fact, furthering one of my own stated goals: that Mrs. M. should feel just that pride. When I did sometimes try to get her to concentrate on the worldly pleasures she could still enjoy, she told me I was not understanding, which was true. What I had to do was not interfere with her own adaptive processes.

I decided that I could best help her by continuing to support her sense of herself as valuable and beautiful, but I did try to stress the internal subjective experience of that, feeling that the fragility of the superficial narcissistic self-evaluation could easily shatter. I had to constantly remind myself that what I was concerned about was not that such a shattering would lead to self-destruction. Volitional self-destruction was her plan, and if she did not carry it out she would suffer an inevitable destruction of her "self" that would be out of her control and terribly cruel. I cannot speak to the physical pain she would have endured, but the emotional agony would have been indescribable. What I had to concern myself with was that if her narcissistic shield was broached, she would, one way or another, still die, but with great shame and terrible unhappiness. My mandate was to maintain her confidence and pride.

Sometimes, of course, she did speak of fear and anger. She was cheated, she felt cheated, she was too young to die, she would never see a grandchild, and she was very scared. At such times I could provide a service that, painful as it was, was still more syntonic for me; I could give her a place to ventilate feelings, agree that she was cheated, and hold fast to my admiration of her. When she expressed anger at and envy of me, I was able to accept and sympathize with the feelings and acknowledge their realistic basis.

Often, however, she needed me to listen as she worked out her scenario. She seemed to feel so useful, and I think, at this time, one of the reasons she rebelled against palliative care was that it threatened the defensive use of her positive self-evaluations. If she was lulled into a temporary sense of physical security, she feared she could lose control of her destiny. I think, too, that her almost cheerful mood reflected the tendency to euphoria that can be seen when a self-destructive enactment is being planned by a neurotic patient. In this case, however, it seemed to be functioning as a kind of analgesic (perhaps for us both), and I believed it best simply to accept it—quite the opposite of the therapeutic decision I would make under other circumstances.

All this was occurring during a holiday season. Mrs. M. gave two major parties that she reported enjoying tremendously, focusing one on honoring a particular professional achievement by her husband. I should note here that she reported that her husband knew her plans for suicide and understood her feelings. She had great confidence in him, she said, but she counted on my professional discretion in any case. At this time, she did not tell me when she expected to carry out her plans.

After some months of this situation, Mrs. M. came to an appointment and requested a straight chair rather than the softer one usually used by patients. She said her back hurt rather badly; she thought she had strained it. She was obviously physically uncomfortable. The same thing happened at our next session, and she spoke of having to cancel dinner plans the night before because of pain. At this session she also described, in greater detail than I had ever heard, her own mother's last years as she declined from Alzheimer's disease, stressing over and over how her mother's personality had changed—"it wasn't her at all," and "she must have been so lonely, not recognizing anyone, me . . ."

I tried to help her express her fear of loss of herself as she knew herself and of being alone. It seemed clear to me that she feared not physical death but emotional destruction; not the aloneness of death but the aloneness of dying if she should have to endure that process in an alien mental state, without awareness of her family, whom she wanted near her—for whatever complex reasons—as she died.

Further, death for her would be not physical destruction, which was about to occur while she was alive, but rather an opportunity for a new beginning, a new chance for self-restitution and perfection. For her, the wish to die included a wish to begin again.

We spoke of aloneness, and she rather hostilely told me that I knew so little, that I could not feel her physical pain, which was increasing; when she left my office she would simply go home to bed—that was her effort for the day. What, she asked, could I know of that? She was quite angry, but then abruptly said, albeit still annoyed, that I would probably never know how much it meant to her that she really could say to me whatever she wanted. Sometimes I sounded stupid, but she knew I was trying. She went on to express a sense of missing her mother, suddenly highlighting, I think, a transference cause for her anger. I said she had granted me a privilege by being so honest and by sharing so much with me.

Since I was about to take a short vacation, Mrs. M. left the office wishing me a good trip and confirming our next appointment. I later realized that she was actually giving me a combination of a gift of reassurance and an assault on my presumption that there would surely be a "next appointment."

The evening I returned I received a telephone call telling me that Mrs. M. had died the day before. As a measure of my own conflict, it is noteworthy that I struggled with whether or not to go to the funeral, a conflict that primarily involved my own denial since my presence would hardly affect my patient; yet the quality of the struggle was as though it might. I did, in fact, attend, for my own sake, of course.

I later learned the details surrounding her death. Mrs. M., with her husband, had bought a very beautiful dressing gown. She chose the day, and on that day carefully made herself up, and in her warm, safe, beautiful bedroom, her "favorite place," her "safe cocoon," near to her husband and daughter, she had taken her pills. Perhaps she had found her way to experience what Eissler (1955) calls the "reawaken[ing of] the primordial feeling of being protected by a mother [by means of which] the suffering of the dying can be reduced to a minimum" (p. 119). I was told that Mrs. M. left long, loving letters to her family and that her death was as she had planned it. I also received a call from a family member with a message she had left for me, thanking me for being so much help to her. I responded to the caller, as I had to her, that it had been a privilege.

NOTE

1. This chapter was presented at a scientific meeting of the New York Freudian Society on October 2, 1992, and as part of a discussion panel at the December 1991 meetings of the American Psychoanalytic Association. It was originally published in the *The Psychoanalytic Study of the Child 49*, eds. A. J. Solnit, P. B. Neubauer, S. Abrams, and A. Scott Dowling (Yale University Press, copyright © 1994 by A. J. Solnit, P. B. Neubauer, S. Abrams, and A. Scott Dowling).

REFERENCES

Bach, S. (1985). *Narcissistic states and the therapeutic process*. New York: Jason Aronson.
Brodsky, B. (1959). Liebestod fantasies in a patient faced with a fatal illness. *International Journal of Applied Psychoanalytic Studies, 40*, 13–16.

Eissler, K. R. (1955). *The psychiatrist and the dying patient.* New York: International University Press.

Freud, S. (1923). *The ego and the id.* S. E., 19.

Gediman, H. (1981). On love, dying together and Liebestod fantasies. *Journal of the American Psychoanalytic Association, 29*, 607–630.

Jones, E. (1911). On "dying together"—with special reference to Heinrich von Kleist's suicide. In *Essays on Applied Psycho-Analysis.* New York: International University Press.

Norton, J. (1968). Treatment of a dying patient. *Psychoanalytic Study of the Child, 18*, 541–560.

Pollack, G. H. (1974). Manifestations of abnormal mourning: Homicide and suicide following the death of another. *Annual of Psychoanalysis., 4*, 225–249.

———. (1975). On mourning immortality and utopia. *Journal of the American Psychoanalytic Association, 23*, 334–362.

Roose, L. (1969). The dying patient. *International Journal of Applied Psychoanalytic Studies, 50*, 385–396.

Sandford, B. (1957). Some notes on a dying patient. *International Journal of Applied Psychoanalytic Studies, 38*, 158–165.

Wald, C. (1957). Suicide as a magical act. *Bulletin of the Menninger Clinic, 21*, 91–98.

Chapter Nine

Guidelines to Live by and Rules to Break

John W. Barnhill, MD

Serious illness complicates psychotherapy. Medical urgency can also focus the treatment, highlight previously covered-over material, and allow for significant growth in a short period of time. In order to minimize the difficulties and encourage effectiveness, therapists who work with sick and dying patients must be willing to demonstrate an unusual amount of clinical flexibility, including breaking a few psychoanalytic rules.

This chapter will focus on Amy Barrett,[1] a thirty-nine-year-old woman whom I met while she was in the process of being diagnosed with breast cancer. I treated her while she was in and out of the hospital for the ensuing year. The focus of the chapter will be on 1) her reaction to the illness; 2) my and the medical team's reaction to her illness; 3) interventions that are unusually "medical" for an analyst; and 4) reactions and interventions that are outside the norm or are potentially controversial. Additional topics will include ways in which individual psychodynamic treatment and countertransference are affected by severe pain, regressions, hostile projections, family involvement, and inevitable death.

HISTORY OF PRESENT ILLNESS

Amy Barrett was a thirty-nine-year-old woman who was in her usual state of robust physical and emotional health until she was hospitalized following a traffic accident. A breast lump and axillary lymphadenopathy were found on routine exam, and the primary medical team anticipated that the work-up would yield a cancer diagnosis. During that evaluation phase, the primary medical team called my psychiatric consultation-liaison (CL) service in order to help anticipate the patient's reaction if the news happened to be bad. As is customary, two members of my CL team—a medical student and a psychiatric resident—were called to do the initial assessment prior to my involvement. They hesitated, questioning whether we could "anticipate" someone's reaction to an unmade diagnosis and wondering what they should suggest to the patient was the pretext for the consultation. I suggested to them that they introduce themselves and simply ask if there was anything we could do. I also suggested that they explain that as far as we knew, no one had additional information about her diagnosis.

Prior to even seeing the patient, I had many questions. Why would the medical team call us when there didn't seem to be anything wrong with the patient? What were the characteristics of this patient that precipitated the unusual behavior? Was there a specific patient/staff interaction that led to this unusual request, or—most likely—did this young, well-educated patient induce unusually strong identifications along with feelings of guilt, helplessness, or sadness in the treating team? Since I don't treat the primary medical team, I can only guess at those answers, but there is usually something particular about the patient who elicits an unusual staff reaction. More practically, however, I wondered whether we should simply have refused to do the consult until after the diagnosis was made and a more routine consult question elicited.

My misgivings were somewhat moot, however, since she was unavailable to my team until I was ready to see the patient. Some demographic information was, however, available from the chart.

PERSONAL HISTORY

Ms. Barrett had been a very successful student and had supported herself through writing since graduating from an elite college. At the time of the hospitalization, she lived in New York City and was a journalist for a well-known publication. Ms. Barrett's parents had divorced when she was nineteen, and she had no siblings. She described her mother as "decent and kind in a Presbyterian sort of way," while her physician father was "an ass but otherwise likable." They lived in a different region of the country ("about 1,000 miles from here physically, and 10,000 miles psychologically").

Ms. Barrett was in a long-term relationship with Jane Simmons, who was an attorney for a large law firm. Both of them had been open about their homosexuality since their early twenties and, while Ms. Barrett's parents had initially been disappointed, they had been accepting of her homosexuality for over a decade.

Psychiatric and Substance Abuse History: Sporadic alcohol and marijuana, but no known history of abuse. No history of psychotherapy or psychiatric illness.

Family Psychiatric History: None known.

Family Medical History: Two of Ms. Barrett's relatives had died from cancer: her grandmother at age fifty-two from breast cancer and her uncle at age forty-nine from prostate cancer.

Medical History: No substantive history. Ms. Barrett had never had a mammogram.

Mental Status Exam: Ms. Barrett was a thin woman who was alert, cooperative, coherent, and engaging. She wore a hospital gown and appeared her stated age. She had mild bruising from the traffic accident. She made good eye contact. She spoke clearly and rapidly. She was worried but her affect was full range. She denied psychosis and suicidality. Her insight and judgment were intact.

INITIAL SESSIONS

I met Ms. Barrett in her hospital room. Another patient and her visitor sat nearby, on the other side of a thin curtain. Seated next to me were a psychiatry resident, a medical student, and Ms. Simmons, her girlfriend, who had declined my invitation to leave the room.

As soon as I sat down, Ms. Barrett wondered why psychiatry was called when she wasn't especially upset. She asked, "So are you guys the angels of death? Surely they don't send in psychiatry when the news is going to be good."

Her girlfriend interjected, "Play nice."

I smiled and told them, "It's a good point. I don't really know why we were called so early, especially when you seem to be doing okay. As for the results of the tests, we haven't seen final reports, and even if we had seen them, we wouldn't be the ones to outline the results or the treatment plan."

Ms. Barrett nodded and said, challengingly, "You use the word 'final,' which means you've seen the preliminary reports, so I guess I should assume that the news won't be great."

"I misspoke about the word 'final,'" I said. "I really don't know the results of any of your tests, though I can see why you'd guess that they'd call us only if the news was bad. But if that's the case, they haven't told us either."

"This is a waste of time," Ms. Barrett responded.

After a brief silence, Ms. Simmons said, "Since we're up in the air about the diagnosis, why don't we take a rain check. Maybe you could come back tomorrow." Ms. Barrett turned on the television, and we left.

By the next day, I had received several phone calls. Two were from hospital colleagues who knew the patient and asked what I'd done to make her angry; one suggested, half jokingly, that irritating an investigative journalist may not be the best career move. A third was from my psychiatry resident saying that the bone scan indicated metastatic cancer. A fourth call was from a good friend of mine; she had dated the patient while they were in college and was friendly with the couple; she added that they wanted me to return as soon as possible, preferably without students.

When I returned the next day, both Ms. Barrett and I were alone. She was very quick to point out that I was either a liar or incompetent, that I'd not brought my henchmen this time because I didn't want to be embarrassed, and that widespread mets meant that nothing could be done for her. Her tone had changed, however, and I felt that she wanted me to engage rather than leave. I pointed out that she was obviously very smart but that I really hadn't known about the mets. I'd not brought my trainees because I'd thought she wanted to meet alone. And, finally, I pointed out that the presence of mets does not mean that nothing can be done. She smiled and said, "No need to get defensive. I was horrible yesterday, but I won't bite today. Maybe you should just start asking about my childhood."

I present dialogue in order to give some flavor of the interaction. Criticisms, humor, and existential angst were intermingled throughout the therapy, and she seemed to need the banter to create a connection and to maintain a comfortable interpersonal distance.

During that second session, Ms. Barrett outlined a strikingly successful professional career. She emphasized that she was worried but hopeful, that everyone in the gay community knew her to be tough and resilient. She had always been independent but would consider a referral, preferably to a lesbian therapist. She also said that she might break up with Jane; she wasn't feeling especially close to her lately and added, jokingly, that cancer would make her a hot commodity among "stray co-dependent lesbians." My goals during these interactions were twofold: the first was to develop an alliance, and the second was to try to empathize with her situation, an effort that meant bypassing her humor and intellectualized defenses and working toward greater understanding. These efforts felt, at times, opposed. For example, banter seemed to enhance the alliance but did not immediately help in the pursuit of empathy. Similarly, a stolid focus on her point of view was sometimes meaningful and sometimes discomfiting to her.

We met several times during this hospitalization. Just prior to her discharge, we met for what I assumed would be her final session. She said she had a few questions: Should she stay involved with Jane? Should she quit her job or take a leave of absence? Should she make a "cancer announcement" or let people find out for themselves? Should she outline the progress of her treatment in a series of articles or would that be too exhibitionistic and maudlin? But would that at least keep the medical team on its toes, or would they become too wary and worried? Should she start medications in case she gets depressed? Was I gay? Would I "puhleeze" call her Amy and not Ms. Barrett? Would I see her in psychotherapy following discharge?

I considered and would later discuss all of her questions with her, but the important question was whether we should work together after she was discharged. The decision to take her into treatment was complicated by several factors: she knew a good friend of mine and would, therefore, potentially have unusual access to my personal life. Anonymity is a cardinal psychoanalytic principle, but it is primarily useful for transference-focused treatments that allow for the freer development of certain kinds of fantasies. Its importance has—in my opinion—been overstated both in terms of its importance and its practicality (the alert patient picks up a lot about us just by how we talk, act, and decorate our offices), and, anyway, my academic web page revealed more about me than my mentors would ever have revealed. Further, we had developed an alliance based at least partly on my relatively open stance about information, and that alliance had prompted her to seek treatment.

My decision about taking her into treatment was complicated by several other factors. She had definitely stated that she preferred a referral to a lesbian therapist, and their first appointment was already set up. I'd long before decided, however, that patients need not work with demographically identical therapists. While overlapping backgrounds and an intimate knowledge of relevant developmental and life issues could be useful, demographically similar therapeutic dyads could also lead to "blind spots" in the treatment. Further, such a perspective would relegate me to only working with WASP heterosexuals, which would be a suboptimal professional decision in the melting pot of Manhattan. Nevertheless, she had already made it clear that almost all of her friends were gay men and women, and she tended to think straight people were some combination of boring, small-minded, misguided, or imperceptive. I later learned that she believed that to be true of most gay people as well, but I didn't know that until weeks later.

Another important factor related to her poor prognosis. As a CL psychiatrist, I was accustomed to working with the terminally ill, but I recognized that it might be especially painful to care for her in her final months. I also viewed it as a precious opportunity, so I was ready for that commitment.

I was more concerned that her tendencies toward verbal aggression and behavioral withdrawal would undermine the treatment. At the same time, I viewed her as perceptive, smart, and witty, and I felt I could more or less keep up with her. Time was an additional factor. I was already getting pressure from home to work fewer hours, but I rationalized that she could easily afford my full fee and that she had complete schedule flexibility.

While the decision was, perhaps, complicated by those factors, the actual decision was made when she listed a series of questions that underlined her cloaked dependency and then asked for help.

OUTPATIENT TREATMENT

The ensuing months were marked by various cancer treatments and debilitation. She took a leave of absence from work. She increasingly restricted her circle of friends. She broke up with Jane. She complained of bony pain and poor concentration. Her mother moved into her apartment. All of the treatment regimens appeared to be ineffective.

During these months, we scheduled twice-weekly sessions, but she frequently did not come to my office because of fatigue or pain. She would, however, call at the appointed time and talk for a few minutes. The sessions were sometimes chatty, but they often focused on regrets, losses, and guilt over squandered opportunities. She was particularly upset that she had never had a child but was at least glad that she hadn't brought a child into the world if he or she were going to be an orphan.

SECOND HOSPITALIZATION

As her condition worsened, Amy was admitted for a complex treatment that included a bone marrow transplant. She asked if I would visit her daily in the hospital. I hedged and said I would come as often as I could. She was ultimately hospitalized for three months with a series of complications. As she became sicker and less able to care for herself, she gradually refused all visitors except her mother.

Varieties of discomfort and pain intensified through much of the hospitalization, and she began to use increasing doses of opioids. A core dilemma developed: she was either undermedicated for tests (leading to pain upon movement, test refusals, and criticisms of the staff) or over sedated (leading to daytime sleep, nighttime insomnia, and further criticisms). This incident pain and pseudo addiction led to accusations of opioid abuse by the staff and accusations of malpractice by the patient. We were able to create a regimen that included a standing dose of an opioid with a moderate half-life as well as an as-needed opioid with a short half-life that she could use prior to tests. This was useful.

Amy became preoccupied with the possibility that God was targeting her. She didn't know exactly what she had done, but she frequently discussed why God would hurt her so much. She also wondered why the staff was so lazy, withholding, and mean. She explained that she refused visitors because it took too much energy to entertain them, and she didn't want them getting brownie points for visiting their dying friend.

Amy was often angry with virtually everyone, then, but not at me or at her mother. Predictably, her hostile projections alienated the nurses, social workers, and doctors, and they did indeed begin to avoid her and provide care that was less thorough than might be expected. Further, they then began to call me whenever (or at least it seemed like whenever) she burst into tears or needed to sign an informed consent.

During this period, I had mixed therapeutic success. I tried to clarify God's role in her illness, specifically exploring whether she viewed God as an entity that inflicted pain or as an entity that might be especially comforting in times of pain. She suggested that I "go back to Unitarian Sunday School, since your God may be cute as a puppy but I'm here getting fucked." In exploring the details of her enmity towards the staff, she detailed many minor "errors"—such as medications being given fifteen minutes late—and dismissed my suggestion that fifteen minutes wouldn't be seen as an error. I even pointed out that the stress of the illness, pain, opioids, and hospitalization had really worn her down and seemed to have led her to more black-and-white thinking than was usual for her; while her mother and I had escaped so far, perhaps she was being too tough on the staff and God, since I didn't think either of them had it out for her. This effort led to irritated sarcasm and fatigue.

My central strategy in dealing with regression, distortion, and projection was not to make clarifications (i.e., to argue with her) but rather to explore what had led her to getting into this situation. My underlying aim was to make sense of relevant experiences, talents, failures, and successes in an effort to return her to her previous trajectory, using her customary defenses. This led to episodic discussions of work, writing, friends, girlfriends, New York, money, and disappointments, and, when successful, appeared to be reliably accompanied by a greater capacity for resilience, humor, patience, and openness to friends.

Through these sessions, we gradually developed a thesis that much of her professional and personal motivation stemmed from feeling misunderstood as a child, relating to her being homosexual and to having parents whom she felt never "got" her. She believed that her efforts at writing and investigation were related to her curiosity about others, her hatred of boredom, and her hope that someone else would work hard to get to know her. Girlfriends had been her potential salvation, but they had consistently disappointed her by either being too needy/intrusive, too distant/unloving, or both. She was aware that she got very dependent, embarrassed at the degree to which she had become dependent upon her mother and me (but was somewhat relieved that we were both stuck in our roles and wouldn't tell her friends), and grudgingly aware that she had broken up with Jane because of the fear of and need for dependency (but she wouldn't change her mind and refused to even talk to her during the hospitalization).

Most of our sessions did not, however, feature such insights, partly because medical complications, pain, and opioids contributed to cognitive and emotional difficulties that reduced the effectiveness of psychotherapy. In addition, therapeutic effort was complicated by time issues (we met frequently but scheduling was complicated by my day's unpredictability and her often being either unavailable or asleep) and money issues (the breakup with Jane—who was a law firm partner—coincided with Amy's inability to work, so the fee dropped significantly throughout the treatment).

Amy did gradually stabilize, however, and was eventually discharged. The above summary of the second hospital stay does not elaborate on family work (I met regularly with the patient and her mother and twice with her and both parents—she ultimately decided, for example, that her father wasn't as big an ass as she'd thought). It does not elaborate on ways that she conformed to the so-called "difficult patient," ways in which the medical teams shied away from her, and relevant hospital dynamics. I also do not greatly explore her dependency issues, her breakup with Jane just when she vitally needed a partner, her idealization of her mother and me, and the fantasied relationship between her physician father and me. I do not write much about my feelings about her, though I think it's clear that she was exasperating, endearing, and funny. I don't mention the extent to which I revealed to her my reactions, beliefs, and history, though I was consciously aware of being relatively transparent (e.g., being explicit about my views on homosexuality and the current president), directive (e.g., when she was regressed in the hospital, I told her to be nice to nurses, call friends, and write in her journal), and organizing (e.g., regardless of the frequency of calls from her or her proxies, I would clarify that I would come to her room for fifteen to twenty minutes, most days of the week). I do not explore the bias that might have led to my selecting this particular patient for VIP treatment (e.g., I saw her often for almost a year, when, ordinarily, I would see her once or twice, the residents would see her as needed, and none of us would treat her as an outpatient). I do not discuss much about medications, the possibility of delirium, breast cancer genetics, or how her cancer complications were challenged by medical fund of knowledge. I also do not explore my thoughts about how her psychosexual development might interlace with her hypomania and isolation. Finally, I do not discuss the evaluation and possible treatment of psychiatric disorders related to anxiety or depression.

Following discharge, Amy flew to her hometown to live with her mother. I called three times and left messages on her mother's answering machine. She died a month later. I sent cards to both parents but didn't again speak to them. Weeks later, I returned from a vacation to find out that I had missed her memorial service in New York.

SUMMARY AND DISCUSSION

As a psychoanalyst and CL psychiatrist, my professional life is guided by sets of professional doctrines that are sometimes in conflict. For example, maintaining relative anonymity encourages the development of a workable, patient-centered transference; even in non-analytic settings, anonymity affords privacy, which—at the least—allows the therapist to work in familiar comfort. In trying to develop a workable and rapid alliance as a CL psychiatrist, however, I frequently highlight similarities or display genuine interest in a patient's hobbies. While likely viewed with suspicion if done during an analytic evaluation, such behaviors are standard fare in the CL world.

With Ms. Barrett, for example, our alliance developed more quickly and deeply as she found out about our shared acquaintances and shared background. The relationship was lopsided in that she talked extensively while I rarely talked about my own feelings or history, but it seemed stabilizing for me to be relatively transparent. Aside from demographic and political tidbits that I assumed we'd share, I also admitted to having gone to a college that I anticipated would lead her to sarcasm. I was also ready to admit to being heterosexual, which I figured might alienate her but which—like the identity of my alma mater—were not deep, dark secrets but rather fairly superficial facts that she could easily find out on her own. I also revealed some of my reactions to her struggling with unsuccessful and painful cancer treatments, but I had some reasons: she had shrugged off all her friends and was only talking to her mother and me. My revelations were intended to underline our connection but also to demonstrate that while I was saddened and upset by her struggles, I wasn't going to abandon her.

Anonymity is related to privacy. While I was primarily trained in a world in which the patient-therapist relationship was as protected as that of the confessor-priest, we held many of our interviews within earshot of other patients and their visitors. Further, I met with and talked to both her parents, and I talked frequently with members of her treating teams. She knew about these discussions and agreed to them, but they contrast dramatically with my typical outpatients, whose multi-year treatments generally include no contact with anyone aside from the patient. Neutrality is another core psychoanalytic guideline. It is a dynamic principle that demands that the analyst nimbly assess and shift his or her perspective to remain equally poised between the ego, id, and superego. Contrasted with suggestion, neutrality is a concept that remains integral to the field even as the structural model of id, ego, and superego has lost its central importance. In regard to Amy Barrett, I made use of suggestion on a regular basis. For example, I frequently found myself reminding her that yelling at hospital staff or relatives was not likely to yield the sorts of results that she was seeking and that her sense of isolation might be improved if she would return the phone calls that kept pouring in despite her failure to ever pick up the phone.

Finally, analytic therapists are expected to maintain a perspective of abstinence in which they refrain from seeking gratification from their patients. Like the other analytic guidelines, abstinence is a virtue that is more often recognized in a dramatic breach than in a typical, modest transgression. For example, it is clearly counterproductive for the therapist to focus the treatment in ways that do not help the patient but rather gratify the therapist. Leaving aside obvious transgressions related to sex and money, typical abuse of the abstinence guideline might include the therapist guiding the therapy into topics that the therapist finds entertaining.

In regard to Amy, I felt something of a balancing act. I wanted to listen to her perspective and to empathize with her lost opportunities, her physical discomfort, and her sense that her future was dramatically being cut short. I consciously worked to maintain that perspective. At the same time, she was not someone who wanted the focus to always be on her problems. She wanted to be entertaining and smart, and she wanted to know whether I was enjoying our interaction. A somber sense of abstinence would, I think, have been counterproductive, so I made an effort to regularly engage in the sort of banter that might have been defensive and distancing and might have broken the abstinence rule but without which she might have been unable to continue in treatment.

Similar flexibility was also useful in regard to schedules and fees. I neither charged for missed sessions nor mandated a rigorous therapy schedule. Some of my rationale was practical in that—in contrast to when I was in full-time practice—I do have scheduling flexibility and have plenty of activities to occupy me during cancelled sessions.

In retrospect, my "breaking" these rules might have contributed to a mistake. As I have outlined, we met frequently during that second hospitalization, and I largely replaced what had been a large group of friends. When Amy returned to her home many miles away, I was startled that she and her mother didn't return my calls. The effort to reach her could be seen as a countertransference enactment in that I was behaving more proactively than is typical of me, since, generally, I let the patient decide whether or not she wants to speak to me.

That potential enactment didn't worry me, however. I was more worried by my failure to anticipate a piece of behavior that should have been easy to predict. By viewing myself as her strong ally, I didn't anticipate that she would do to me what she had done to all of her friends: abandon them before she could get abandoned. The same intensity of connection that had been—I think—particularly helpful during her hospitalization likely contributed to my failure to anticipate with the patient and her mother that she might feel obliged to abandon me when she returned home. By not anticipating this behavior, I lost the opportunity to be helpful during her final weeks, which were, I worry, ravaged by pain, confusion, and a sense of failure. At the same time, I was also aware that my own powers to help were limited, that Amy and her mother had plenty of evidence that I would respond to their call, and that those final weeks might not have been improved by a few phone calls from me.

In summary, then, our work together was incomplete but still, I think, useful. Through session after session, we were able to discuss her inactivity, physical wasting, and crescendos of pain, social isolation, and our shared sense that our options were limited. While we molded some analytic principles to fit the situation, we did follow the core analytic perspective of spontaneous, benevolent curiosity. Even during her periods of mild confusion and harsh humor, she seemed significantly calmed by this ongoing effort at connection. In the end, of course, she died. I hope I was able to provide some comfort during her final year, but I am confident that my ongoing efforts at understanding what goes into therapy make it possible for me to continue to work with challenging patients like Amy Barrett.

NOTE

1. The patient's name and some of her demographic information have been altered to protect her privacy.

Chapter Ten

"Titration of Psychotherapy for Patient and Analyst"

Alison C. Phillips, MD

This case presentation highlights many of the principles that are recommended for a flexible psychoanalytic psychotherapy for cancer patients facing death. The analyst maintains a highly flexible approach regarding technique attuned to the patient's needs. Accordingly, the analyst refrains from fully analyzing resistances, and a commonsense approach to defenses is adopted to permit optimal coping. Powerful countertransferences stemming from identification with the patient, survivor guilt, and feelings of helplessness are noted and managed. As the author reflects on this treatment she can not be certain as to the effect of her decision to not interpret the patient's resistances. Were they in the service of optimal adaption and coping or were they a function of counter transference? I think both.

Susan and I dosed her psychotherapy like her chemotherapy. For much of the fourteen months that I treated Susan, we met on an every-other-week schedule alternating with her chemotherapy, but she also took breaks. Together, I believe that we enacted a shared belief that, like chemotherapy, psychotherapy had the potential to help and the potential to weaken her needed defenses. Early on, Susan informed me that, similar to chemotherapy, she experienced "aftereffects" of psychotherapy with me. I did too.

Susan particularly moved me. A beloved health care worker and devoted mother with strong commitments to family, friends, and work, she was a self-described "glass half-full" person. I felt privileged to witness Susan face her diagnosis and treatment of metastatic cancer with remarkable strength and grace. But treating Susan also pushed me to confront unbearably painful feelings and fears, to question the goals and structure of psychoanalytically informed therapy for patients with late-stage, incurable cancer, and to reflect on Susan's oscillation between disavowal and acknowledgement of her cancer and the parallel enactment of this oscillation between us.

From the start, Susan's ambivalence about coming for therapy, as well as the extent of her connection with others, was apparent. When I asked, in the first session, what brought her in, she replied, "I'm here because I have a friend who cares very much about me." This friend was also trying to come to terms with Susan's recent diagnosis of late-stage, metastatic cancer and to be as helpful as possible. Though Susan had briefly been in psychotherapy only once before, she impressed me with her capacity for insight and reflection. She described herself as happy and grateful for the life she had, which included a close-knit and very supportive family of origin, three "wonderful" children, a strong network of friends, and a job she loved. She remarked at a later date that she would not be coming to see me were it not for "the cancer."

Although I didn't articulate it as such, in retrospect my ambivalence about treating Susan was also present from the start. After our first session, I remember thinking as she left, "She will bear this, but I'm not sure if I can." Susan didn't cry easily. I don't cry easily either, but in those early months of treatment, there were times with her when I started to feel panicky that if I started to cry I would not be able to stop. I found myself worrying about crying when she was not, because I didn't want to burden her with having to take care of me, too, something she felt acutely with her family and friends. I wondered, though, whether I held more of the painful affect in our sessions, and if this was a reflection of Susan's need to separate herself from her sorrow.

Susan and I had many overt characteristics of our lives in common, from our age, ethnic background, and number and age of our children to our sensibilities and life values. I think that these shared features intensified my identification with her and made it much harder for me to defensively deny that I was just as likely to develop cancer as she, and also heightened my experience of survivor guilt. It was, in fact, the moments when she spoke of leaving her children that brought tears for both of us. But there was more to my countertransferential experience with Susan. Something about her grace, acceptance, and capacity for empathy rendered her words extremely poignant and compelling for me. I often felt that she was showing me how to preserve and experience life in the shadow of death. I think, on some level, I imagined that she was handling her diagnosis, medical treatment, and fears of death far better than I ever would. I wonder now, though, whether my "in awe of her" countertransference interfered with my ability to confront some of her ambivalence about psychotherapy.

Susan often reflected on how her experience of time had changed since her diagnosis, and the way that cancer had "super-highlighted" life for her. I too noticed a change in my experience of "time" in our psychotherapy. In contrast to most therapy and analysis where significant time is spent looking back at the past and imagining a future, Susan and I focused acutely and intensely on the present. Well into our work together, I became aware that I knew only the broad brushstrokes of Susan's early life. I knew that she had grown up in an intact family, with parents who were, and continued to be, loving and attentive to her. But it was a family that never spoke the language of emotion, and Susan had always felt the expectation that she be stable and "fine." Her mother was a model of stoicism, never giving in to emotional or physical distress. Even her father, the more emotionally accessible of the two, questioned why Susan needed to see me. Susan had approached other major challenges in her life with the stance of "picking myself up and carrying on."

Susan reported that she had always been more concerned about other people than herself. As an experienced caregiver, she was far less comfortable being on the receiving end. She had never been at ease in the spotlight, so the spotlight of having cancer presented a real challenge for her. "I've become aware of the power of me," she told me. While she didn't want to avoid talking about her cancer, she wished to reassure people that she was "okay," in part to relieve the fear and intense concern she read in their reactions, but she also wanted people to engage with her, not just focus on her cancer. Desperately wanting to live her life as normally as possible and for others to treat her as normally as possible, she struggled to maintain a sense of separateness from her cancer for herself and others. But when she began to lose her hair secondary to the chemotherapy, this more overt physical sign threatened her sense of separateness from her cancer. Surprised at how much losing her hair upset her she said, "It's not that I'm vain, it's just that it becomes so obvious and I don't want people to feel awkward around me."

Susan frequently used the words "fine" and "normal" to describe how she was feeling to the people in her daily life and to me. We explored the "disconnect" she felt, particularly in the early months following her diagnosis, between feeling "fine" and knowing that she was seriously ill. Like losing her hair, coming to therapy forced her to confront this disconnect and put her in a difficult bind. She was committed to living as normally as possible in the time she had remaining, To her, this meant focusing on day-to-day activities and concerns, maintaining a positive attitude, and minimizing the time she spent worrying about her illness and the future. However, in therapy she inevitably ended up focusing on her cancer and "negative thoughts" about dying and the suffering she imagined this would entail for her family. She worried that letting in negative, fearful thoughts might threaten her functioning. However, she and I both knew that she also needed and wanted a place where she could explore and express her sadness and fear without feeling that she was burdening a loved one or having to take care of their feelings. She informed me that she frequently contemplated canceling our sessions. Sometimes the "little voice inside me that says this is important," convinced her otherwise, but at other times it was not enough to overcome her desire to avoid the prospect of feeling the fear and pain. She told me, "I would never lay this on anyone else, I don't know how to. With you, I know it stops here." She paused. "And?" I question. "You'll be all right without me; I'm not sure others will be."

So, despite knowing that Susan was not psychologically fragile, I felt acutely aware of the tension between helping her give voice to her deepest fears and pain, and not wanting to push it too far, to take away her means of coping through this difficult time. She experienced a similar conflict with her children. At one point, the father of one of her teenage son's friends was diagnosed with cancer shortly before Susan died. When Susan's son became very upset and angry, she wondered how much of his reaction was precipitated by his fears about her. "I didn't know how much of me he was putting in the picture. It was devastating. I didn't want to avoid it, but I didn't want him to be pulled deeper. I felt so helpless, I wanted to say to him that it's different for me, but I can't." She didn't know how to help him. On the one hand, she believed that she needed to prepare him for her death, and on the other hand, she feared that she might be forcing too much pain and suffering on him before it was necessary.

About eight months into our work together, we increased the frequency of sessions to once per week. When, in one of these sessions, she described her experience of the increased frequency as "exploring this thing I can't see, feel, or touch," I imagined that she was speaking about both her cancer and about her unconscious. After I acknowledged her mixed feelings about this kind of exploration, she associated to the meaning she now assigned to bodily aches and pains. She feared that any pain meant the cancer had grown or spread to that area of her body, and was frustrated with "not knowing." She concluded, though, "I suppose I don't want to know." Then, she began to describe a trip to the beach over the past weekend. In the car, her daughter pronounced that she wanted to get married one day on a beach. At that moment Susan was struck by the agonizing thought, "I won't be there." In the car and then in this session with me, she allowed herself to feel the fear and sadness of leaving her children. "It's not for me that I'm concerned, it's for them. I am the glue of everything." Then she reflected, "I suppose that when you can put aside the negative thoughts, and put in positive thoughts, that's what's called the fight. But it's not a fair fight." She went on to imagine what life would be like for her family after she dies. In this particularly difficult session, Susan revealed that coming weekly made it harder for her to compartmentalize her "negative thoughts." After this session, she decided to take a several-month break from therapy. It coincided with a break from chemotherapy that her oncologist had recommended because she was experiencing severe side effects.

At this and at other points during our work, I struggled with how much to explore and interpret what would be classically seen as resistance. Interestingly, she never cancelled because of illness. Rather, she generally cancelled because of a commitment that arose for work or her children. In a traditional sense, she was canceling to avoid confronting painful thoughts and feelings about her illness and to avoid feelings of dependency on me, which heightened her sense of helplessness and vulnerability. But looked at with a different, more flexible lens crucial to the treatment of patients with late-stage or terminal illness, she was also choosing to seize those aspects of her life that provided her with the most meaning and sense of normalcy. "I love the work I do, and the people I work with. And it's a distraction. So if I have to choose between talking with you about dying or working with six-year-old. . . . I choose the distraction."

As our work together continued, Susan did begin to take more of an interest in the origins of her thoughts, behavior, and defensive style. She began to wonder whether a form of "denial" interfered with her seeking treatment before her cancer was so far advanced. She hadn't been feeling "herself" for a long time, but dismissed various physical symptoms as too minor to warrant seeking treatment. She was never one to go to the doctor or miss work unless she was very ill. "I've never been one to complain, I've always been very accepting of what life brings." Now, she started to question this stance: "Maybe if I had been less accepting, I would have gone to a doctor sooner." She noticed that she had been asserting herself more, and in sessions became more interested in why she "didn't allow myself to act for so long in my life."

On her way to a session toward the end of our work together, Susan stopped for a hot chocolate. "I would never have allowed myself to have a hot chocolate in the past. Maybe a plain coffee or a skim milk latte," she confided. She spoke about wanting me to see a fuller picture of her than her cancer. As she mused about what other people came to explore with me, I imagined that she was telling me that she wanted to have a "normal" psychotherapy, at least some of the time, not just a therapy about dying. I asked whether there might be other aspects of her life that she would like to explore. "There are things to explore . . . I'm just not sure how to start." She looked at me with a tentative smile, anxious and excited about the "chance to really understand myself." "Kind of like allowing yourself hot chocolate," I said. "Yes," she replied, "it sounds so nice, like a luxury." At that moment, I felt excited and hopeful too, but shortly after Susan discontinued treatment with me.

For me, it was an unanticipated and upsetting end. In what was to be her final session with me, she told me that her most recent scan had looked "stable" and that she and her family had settled into a "new kind of normal" in their daily life. She was relieved that other people in her life were treating her more normally as well. Following this session, she left me a message asking to reschedule our next session. However, she did not respond to my return phone calls to reschedule, and after several attempts, I decided not to continue to pursue her. Ultimately, I chose to respect her need to terminate with me in this way, accepting that I could only speculate about why. I recognized that it was a time of relative stabilization of her cancer, which enabled her to achieve a "new normal," a compartmentalization of her cancer that she wanted to maintain for as long as possible. And coming to see me was a constant reminder of her cancer. But I struggled with a mix of sadness, hurt, and doubts about my work with her. Over the ensuing months, I thought of her often, wondering how she was doing and whether she was still alive. I later learned from her friend who had made the original referral that Susan had died about eighteen months after our last session.

Throughout her treatment with me, Susan had titrated the frequency of her sessions with me. But her departure from therapy forced me to consider some difficult questions. In some way, I had imagined that she was optimally titrating her psychotherapy with me so as to "concentrate on living with cancer, not preoccupied with dying of cancer." I think that I wanted to believe that my not pressuring her to come more frequently reflected my attunement to supporting her needed defenses. On further reflection, though, I recognized that perhaps this did not fully account for my role in what I now see as a mutually enacted titration of therapy. As someone who was so sensitive to her effect on others, I wonder whether Susan was reading how moved I was by her, often painfully so, and therefore in part titrating for me. And did I unconsciously collude with her titration because I was unsure how much I could bear? I did know that I anxiously imagined her dying and her funeral. What would it be like? How would I be able to help? How close would she let me be and how close would I allow myself to be?

In the end, Susan chose to leave me in life, while her mind, body and defenses were still intact, instead of in death. Perhaps she imagined sparing us both the witnessing of her deterioration and a good-bye that felt too painful.

I will never know whether it would have been helpful for Susan to come more frequently or whether our work together really did represent an optimal titration of psychotherapy for her at this stage of her life. Susan sometimes questioned whether she was "in denial," a word frequently invoked when evaluating the extent of a cancer patient's acceptance of their illness. Susan was fully compliant with chemotherapy and cancer treatment and was intent on doing whatever she could to fight the battle. She maintained a positive attitude and tried to carry on with her life as fully and "normally" as possible, rarely complaining with any intensity about the debilitating side effects of chemotherapy. In regard to chemotherapy, she told me, "I don't believe it won't work, but I don't believe it will cure me. I've got to believe I have more time." I think, in her question about denial, Susan was speaking to her powerful need to separate herself from the cancer and from the painful feelings that accompanied it. So much of the experience of having incurable cancer felt out of her control. But, she told me, "it is in my power to carry on my day as it was and to harness my negative thoughts."

Instead of the terms "denial" and "acceptance," I think that the concept of an oscillation between disavowal and acknowledgment more aptly captures Susan's psychological experience and the interaction between us. Humphrey Morris has written extensively about his concept that "disavowal/acknowledgment oscillations are at the constitutive core of mental functioning" and describes how they are "inextricably linked," with disavowals being "necessary for getting through life" and "making acknowledgments possible" (unpublished manuscript). This concept seems crucial to an understanding of how someone copes with living in the face of imminent death. Morris notes that Freud originally conceptualized disavowal as a defense against external reality mobilized by a child's ego in the face of perceptions of overwhelming imaginary or real loss. For most people, being given a diagnosis of incurable cancer represents a "real" experience of overwhelming loss.

Disavowing what she knew allowed Susan some comfort and enabled her to maintain hope: she often both knew and didn't know at the same time. For example, when her son had a very intense emotional reaction to the death of his friend's father, I believe she "knew" that his reaction was all about her, but initially she needed to not know this. Susan needed to be able to disavow her inevitable death in order to live. Too much disavowal can lead to a pathological degree of denial; too much acknowledgment of dying can interfere with living.

Clinicians treating patients with cancer are also confronted with the specter of overwhelming loss, with corresponding disavowal/acknowledgment oscillations. It took me some time to realize that Susan and I were engaging in a particular enactment that seemed to reflect our joint disavowal of "time." When we would call to leave messages for each other involving appointment scheduling, neither of us responded promptly. Instead, we both waited a couple of days, which was quite different from my usual attempts to reach patients by the end of the day. It's as if we were both "pretending" that we had all the time in the world to schedule an appointment, that there was no urgency, no life-or-death situation here. I wonder whether our broader titration of psychotherapy ultimately represented a joint disavowal/acknowledgment of each of our fears of death, helplessness, and vulnerability and of the power of psychotherapy.

This treatment highlights many of the essential differences between a psychoanalytic psychotherapy for patients with emotional conflicts and a psychoanalytic psychotherapy for patients with cancer. It is focused primarily in the "here and now" and the issues of life and death are ever present in the therapy. Optimal coping and quality of life are the goals of the therapist. At times, cancer and its consequences are spoken about directly, and at other times, it is disavowed or denied. The patient's defensive style is to temporarily remove herself from the curse of cancer and go about her life in her characteristic manner. The analyst followed the patient's lead, as it was her best judgment that resistance analysis might threaten the stability of the patient. The patient was most comfortable as a caretaker, was stoical, and a glass half-full person who wanted to appear "normal" and would never have considered seeking psychotherapy for herself if it were not for the cancer illness. At the very point when the cancer was stable and the patient was considering a further exploration of herself with the analyst, she retreated to the safety of her lifelong comfort zone. The analyst respected the patient's decision.

Chapter Eleven

Psychotherapy with a Hospitalized Patient Dying of Cancer

M. Philip Luber, MD

This case reveals the multiple roles that the analyst may play as his patient approaches their death. He has individual sessions with the patient as well as interfacing with the family and medical staff. This case also highlights an example of an oncologist's failure to recognize and prepare the patient and family for the imminent death of his patient. Futile toxic chemotherapy is prescribed until the end.

I was asked to see a patient on a medical floor in the hospital to evaluate her depression. The patient, Mrs. F., was a seventy-five-year-old woman with metastatic carcinoma of the colon. After her evaluation, I undertook a four-time-per-week psychotherapy with the patient while she was in the hospital for the three weeks prior to her death. The source of the referral was not the patient's doctor, but rather her daughter. The daughter told me that the request for help was as much for her as for her mother. The daughter felt frightened and depressed about her mother's illness.

I first met with Mrs. F. a few days after her admission to the hospital. Eight years prior to this admission, she was diagnosed with breast cancer, which was successfully treated without serious complications or recurrence. Five years prior to this admission, she was diagnosed with carcinoma of the colon, which also seemed to be successfully treated, without major complications. She had retired in her mid-sixties, and after that led a very active social life, including travel and sports.

Three weeks prior to this admission, she felt weak while playing golf and saw her local doctor in Florida. His work-up revealed a probable recurrence and spread of cancer. Mrs. F. trusted the doctors in New York who had successfully treated her before. She therefore flew to New York to enter the hospital. Further work-up in the hospital revealed that the colon cancer had spread diffusely throughout her body.

When I met the patient, she was lying in bed and looked almost comatose and near death. She was quite thin; the skin of her face pulled tightly over her strong features. Her eyes were shut and she could open them partially, but only with great effort. Speech was difficult; she initially seemed to be mumbling, but careful listening revealed that she was actually quite coherent. The more I spoke with her, the more likely it seemed to me that her obtunded condition was not simply due to physical debilitation or depression; she appeared to be struggling against sedation.

A review of her medications revealed that the intern who admitted her had written orders for whopping doses of sedative-hypnotics. It is not uncommon practice for doctors to over sedate their patients who are dying to reduce their own anxieties. Often this stems from an assumption that the patient will be overwhelmingly depressed about his or her condition, and the doctor cannot bear to hear it.

After speaking to her family and the doctors who knew her, I explained to the medical and nursing staff that Mrs. F. was a highly intelligent woman for whom mental acuity was central to her self-esteem and sense of control. Therefore, it was much more frightening for her to be sedated than to be fully aware of her situation. I recommend that the medication regimen be adjusted to emphasize maximum analgesia and minimum sedation. The house staff carried out my suggestions. Within thirty-six hours of the change in medication, Mrs. F.'s mental status changed dramatically—she became alert, awake, and fully oriented, without any evidence of organicity. She looked forward to our meetings and was eager to talk about her current situation and her past life. She emphasized her difficulty adjusting to such a rapid and dramatic change in her health: she had overcome cancer twice in the past and only three weeks before she had been active and vigorous, playing golf regularly. Now she was seriously ill and confined to the hospital.

The need to evaluate the results of an elaborate metastatic work-up during the first few days of the hospitalization led to the staff's downplaying the likelihood of the obvious poor prognosis. However, once the extent of the spread of the patient's cancer was documented, varying degrees of denial about her imminent death were apparent in both staff and family.

Her husband, a rather passive and dependent man, relied on his wife to organize their daily lives together and had not lived by himself for almost fifty years. Because of the magnitude of the anticipated loss of the "anchor" of his existence, he actively avoided confronting her approaching death. It soon became clear to me that my primary task would be to help the patient prepare for her imminent death. The patient's daughter, a professional woman in her forties, divorced and without children, had a clingy and fearful demeanor. This was in contrast to her dominant and controlling mother. Until recently, she had been in psychotherapy dealing with her difficulty separating from her mother. This dependency on her mother impaired her ability to act in a more assertive manner. She communicated that she was on the verge of being overwhelmed by panic and despair as she faced her mother's condition. The patient's son was a quiet single man in his thirties and, like his father, a marginally successful health professional. He lived in the southwest, and although rather emotionally distant, was appropriately concerned about his mother's health.

As I began working with the patient, I was impressed by the total lack of any kind of coordinated approach by the doctors. The oncologist had recommended a very aggressive treatment approach to the patient without any discussion with the family, the primary internist, or me. The poor prognosis was denied and any discussion of treatment options was avoided. Her oncologist, I learned, was well-known in local medical circles for his unwavering commitment to aggressive treatment with the most advanced tumors in cachectic and dying patients. The patient's internist, a skilled and compassionate woman, was unable or unwilling to rein him in or weigh in with the patient and family. My assessment was that because of the oncologist's character pathology, I could not form an alliance and work with him. I could only try to work around him to help the patient.

Within the limitations imposed by the patient's health and the lack of time and privacy, I gathered as much history as I could. The patient, born in Germany, was the oldest daughter of a middle-class Jewish family. She had always identified with her father, who was an assertive and energetic man. She was somewhat vague in describing her mother, a quieter, less imposing person. She described her younger sister as quiet and shy like her mother. She recalled hardships that accompanied the rise of the Nazis. The first was the loss of their housekeeper when it became illegal for Jews to have gentile domestic help. Shortly thereafter, the patient was forced to give up her studies in one of the health professions. The family then made arrangements to leave Germany and, after a complicated journey, ended up in New York. Several aunts, uncles, and cousins perished in the Holocaust. In this country, the patient got training in a different health field and worked at a job that was not commensurate with her intelligence. Her husband, a passive man, was in a different health discipline, with more potential for income. Mrs. F. pushed him to work harder to develop a successful practice. Her internist described her as strong and admirable, her husband and daughter as weak.

During the initial few days of uncertainty before the extent of the illness and prognosis was known, I explored the patient's feelings about her illness. She sensed that things looked very bad. As I alluded to earlier, the staff avoided all discussion, accepting the treatment advice of the oncologist. I thought that Mrs. F. was the kind of person who would do better by directly confronting facing death. I decided, with some trepidation, to directly broach the subject. I asked her how it felt to be dying. She broke into tears and cried for a long time. I initially worried that I had made a serious error and trashed her defenses. However, it soon became apparent that my anxieties were unfounded. It quickly became clear to the patient, her family, and the staff that she was in better spirits for the rest of the day after the opportunity to express her feelings about dying were offered. My countertransference reaction fears stemmed partly from the fact that I was treating a dying woman who was close in age to my mother. I also initially feared that my direct conversation would make the patient more depressed and suicidal, and ruin my reputation with my medical colleagues,

Mrs. F. cried frequently during her sessions with me. She spoke of her sadness at having to give up the plans she had for the future. She spoke as well about a terrible sense of finality, that she could no longer fantasize about making up in the future for past mistakes or missed opportunities. She said she could not cry in the presence of her family since both she and they required that she continue in a role of stoical strength. In addition to her sadness, she spoke of her anger and bitterness at having to face this painful ordeal. She felt cheated, but this was tempered by a sense of having had a long life with many opportunities for satisfaction. She told me that if she were my age (early forties) when this happened she would be much more bitter and depressed. Later, with some prodding on my part, and after I was away on a long holiday weekend, she acknowledged that she felt envious of my youth and health. She told me she was not particularly religious and had no firm concept of what happened after death; therefore, she had no picture of reunion, reward, or punishment for behavior in life.

She acutely felt the loss of active physical activity and the travel plans which she had to cancel. A small number of friends came to visit her in the hospital, but since she had not lived in this city for a number of years, they were not her closest friends, and that made her sad. One friend brought pictures of grandchildren, which made the patient depressed about not living long enough to have grandchildren of her own. She seemed more down after she received a letter from a niece living in Israel with whom she was close, and whom she and her husband were planning to visit soon. In a session with me she cried about the fact that she would never see her niece again. Her relationship with her niece was particularly poignant because of the strain and disappointment that marked her relationships with her own children.

Her medical care discussions focused on whether or not she would receive chemotherapy for her cancer. It was quite difficult to obtain a realistic picture of what could be expected from such a course of treatment. I was able to ascertain that the consensus of the experts was that chemotherapy in this situation had a 30 percent chance of working, and if it did work, it was likely to prolong the patient's life only two to three months. The debilitating side effects included severe nausea, pain, and weakness. Again, the oncologist continued to press the patient to accept chemotherapy without any discussion with the other doctors involved. He was vague at first but eventually told her that the treatment offered a 30 percent chance of success, but did not tell her what that meant in terms of likely length of survival.

I contacted the oncologist and tried to initiate a discussion with him on how to best present the treatment options to the patient and family. He brushed me aside, declaring in a self-congratulatory way, "Watch me; it's not what you say to the patient, it's how you say it." He meant by this that he was skilled in getting patients to accept his recommendation for aggressive treatment. When other doctors had reservations about the benefit of such aggressive treatment at this point, he said two things: 1) You cannot be in this business and be a nihilist—you've got to try to do something no matter what the odds; and 2) if the chemotherapy did not work there was a good chance it would kill the patient, and that would not be such a bad outcome either. Most of the other doctors involved in the case felt that they would not recommend chemotherapy in this circumstance, but deferred to the oncologist; one specialist told Mrs. F. that he would not recommend chemotherapy if he or his mother were in her position. Initially, I did not share my own opinion, which was that that a course of chemotherapy would probably do more harm than good. Instead, I emphasized that she should not feel pressured by others and that she should decide what was best for her. She obsessed about what to do, flip-flopping back and forth about her decision for the better part of a week.

During one session, Mrs. F. complained about her weakness, loss of functioning, and bleak prospects. She went on to say that she would be better off dead and done with this misery and that sometimes she thought of killing herself. Specifically, she thought of taking an overdose of sedative-hypnotic pills. I told her that there were some things concerning this decision that we needed to discuss; however, it was ultimately her decision. First, I assured her that as her cancer worsened, an analgesic regimen could be instituted to minimize any pain she experienced and that there were other ways to relieve her pain. Second, I posed the question of how she thought her actions would affect her family. She said they would be devastated—filled with confusion and guilt in addition to sadness. I suggested that suicide might be a way of expressing her anger and disappointment to her doctors (including myself) and family for not doing more for her.

Mrs. F. then acknowledged that she felt a lot of bitterness, more than she had wanted to admit. It came as a devastating blow that the doctors could not cure her cancer this time after having beaten cancer twice in the past. She was less comfortable talking about her disappointment that the doctors did not better coordinate her care. After talking about that aspect of her care, she would back away and partially "undo" it. She felt angry that she had to take care of her family even while she was dying. Her husband and her daughter communicated their preoccupation with how her illness affected them rather than her. She was disappointed that they could not give more to her at this critical time. She felt compelled to protect them by not revealing her feelings of sadness and fear; she could only express these in private with me. Her suicidal thoughts became much less frequent and less pressing as we explored these feelings of anger and disappointment.

As the treatment progressed, I became aware of my role as the strong father transference able to face her pain and suicidal wishes. In addition, I think I also functioned as a kind of fantasized idealized son, successful and strong, unlike her own children, who were intelligent, but whose functioning was severely hampered by neurotic conflict. I spoke frequently with her daughter and husband, and less so with her son, who lived in a distant city. I tried to help her husband accept the fact that she was dying and that he had to prepare himself for that reality. I tried to reassure her daughter about the unrealistic nature of some of her fears. I also intervened in her masochistic provocations with the nursing staff. In her panicky and guilt-provoking way, she was demanding and critical of nursing staff. I pointed out to her that her behavior only served to make the nurses angry and less willing to help her mother. I also recommended that she re-enter psychotherapy to deal with her reactions to this stress

Mrs. F. seemed to benefit from the opportunity to look back over her life and discuss pleasurable memories as well as disappointments. She spoke about her disappointment in the passivity of her husband and son, and her daughter's anxious neediness. She continued to debate whether or not to go through with the chemotherapy, tending more and more toward refusing it. I eventually told the patient that if I were in her situation, I would not agree to chemotherapy, and would instead choose a comfortable end-of-life care at home, surrounded by loved ones—but that she had to decide what was right for her. The hospital felt pressure to discharge her if she decided to opt against chemotherapy. The family and social services department looked into the possibility of her going home to Florida, staying with her daughter in the Midwest, or setting up an apartment in New York. However, as she became more debilitated, there were reservations about whether any of these options were feasible. Hospice care was offered as another option.

However, her medical condition rapidly deteriorated, and she became acutely delirious. It was a terrible blow to her that her orientation and memory were impaired, and when I tried to evaluate her cognitive functioning she started repeating, "I'm a vegetable. I'm vegetable." As she became more delirious, she confused "hospice" with a nursing home and thought she was being shipped off because her mind was gone, that she was just a vegetable. There was some indication that in her confusion the experiences and fears of her adolescence in Nazi Germany were revived. I recommended medication to help symptomatically with the delirium. She abruptly decided to go ahead with the chemotherapy. The medical staff then debated whether she had the capacity to make this decision. The question was moot, however, because she died in the hospital before the treatment could be started. It appeared to me that the acute organic brain syndrome led to unrealistic fears about the hospice and accentuated her need for some sense of control as she was losing her most valued attribute, her cognitive ability.

She died at night when I was out of the hospital. I offered to meet with her family after her death; her husband refused, but I met with her daughter and son in my office to help them with the grieving process. Several months later I received a card from the daughter thanking me for the help I had given to her mother and the rest of the family.

Chapter Twelve

Being a Cancer Patient in Analysis while Continuing to Work as an Analyst

Patricia Plopa, PhD

When a man knows he is to be hanged in a fortnight, it concentrates his mind wonderfully.

—Samuel Johnson

I became aware of this quote by Samuel Johnson in a paper by Feinsilver (1998) on "The Therapist as a Person Facing Death: The Hardest of External Realities and the Therapeutic Action." Feinsilver was struggling with colon cancer and continuing to work with his analytic patients. The quote captures how the experience of facing death, while one might wish to avoid or deny it, can also sharpen the mind about what is really important and what needs to be done to survive, if possible, or to resign oneself to death. If it is not traumatic, death anxiety can serve as useful "signal anxiety" in mobilizing internal and external resources to manage adversity with a sense of agency.

I was a practicing psychologist with more than twenty-five years of clinical experience and just beginning my fifth year of training to become a psychoanalyst when the unthinkable (for me) occurred—a cancer diagnosis after a routine mammogram. There had been no breast cancer in my family, not even much cancer, and I had often thought my genetic loading leaned toward cardiac problems, not cancer. My regular, everyday world and vision of my future felt shattered upon learning of the "bad news" (my gynecologist's words) following a biopsy. Before the biopsy and immediately after it, both my gynecologist and the surgeon doing the biopsy had tried to reassure me that the great majority of biopsies yielded negative findings. However, when one hears the "c" word—that is, "cancer"—most think first of death, even when intellectually, one knows that that is not necessarily the trajectory. Yet it is what hits patients' minds, too, most often, even when they don't say it—debilitation, vulnerability, and death—and how will this affect them and their treatment? For the therapist/analyst (I will use the words interchangeably) and the patient, the fear is sharp, and it takes time to settle the mind, to reflect and mourn the sense of safety that has now been lost.

It has now been a number of years since that time, and my fears have diminished, but awareness of mortality is much more of a companion of mine than I assume it would have been had I not had cancer and gone through surgery, chemotherapy, and radiation. Because I was a practicing psychologist and a candidate analyst in training at the time of my diagnosis and treatment, I had some unique pressures as well as supports and opportunities. The pressures included responsibilities of treating patients in psychotherapy in my private practice and patients in four-times-a-week psychoanalysis as part of my analytic training. It also meant being evaluated by supervisors and faculty at the institute where I was being trained. While my supervisors were, thankfully, supportive and helpful, it made for a great deal of personal exposure at a difficult time. I was fortunate to be in my own training analysis, as was required of candidates. The supervision, and especially the analysis, offered an opportunity for reflection and "holding" that might not otherwise been as prominent when one is going through cancer treatment. Without that special "analytic space" and relationship where I could talk about my worst fears and struggles, I could not have continued to work effectively with my patients, tolerating and hearing their worst fears and fantasies about me, the cancer, and their treatments.

What I will attempt to do in the next several pages is to share and explore issues about my experience of working clinically with patients while facing my own illness and fears about death. This will include how my self-disclosure of my cancer, as well as the cancer itself, affected me and my work with patients, as well as the experience and impact of my own analysis and analyst at this time.

At the time of my cancer diagnosis and treatment, I had completed four years of classwork and supervision. I had just received the green light from faculty and supervisors as to the quality of my analytic work, and the major remaining task before applying for graduation was to write a graduation paper. I had already started this project, but changed course and topic after I learned about my cancer. It is part of my personality style to use intellectual mastery as a coping skill in dealing with uncertainty and anxiety. Therefore, besides reading and researching as much as I could tolerate about my type of cancer and the types of treatment for it, I also turned my energies to reviewing the professional literature about illness and cancer in the analyst.

REVIEW

I was interested in what other analysts had written about their experiences with cancer and death, and I discovered that the literature in this area was relatively scarce. Even Freud, who had struggled with cancer of the jaw for the last sixteen years of his life, had not written about the impact of his medical condition on his work and was reluctant to discuss it (Schur, 1972, p. 378). Few analysts wrote about issues of illness in the analyst until 1982, when papers by Abend, Dewald, Halpert, and Silver appeared. In 1990, Schwartz and Silver edited a book, *Illness in the Analyst: Implications for the Treatment Relationship*, which consisted of papers by fourteen analysts addressing personal and clinical implications of life-threatening illnesses and death of the analyst. Many of these authors noted the overall paucity of research and discussion on this topic and suggested it was related to denial and avoidance of exposing countertransference feelings (Abend, 1982; Dewald, 1982; Halpert, 1982). Fieldsteel (1989) surveyed a number of analysts to find out how analysts faced life-threatening illnesses and death. She noted that frequently there was a denial of mortality and an avoidance of addressing the reality of their illness with patients. She reported that some analysts dealt with their illness as a fantasy with patients and she questioned in whose interest it was to treat the idea of an illness as a fantasy.

Much of the early analytic literature did not address analysts' personal experiences of illness and the impact on them and their patients. When analysts did address issues of illness, the emphasis was frequently on the analyst's greater narcissistic self-absorption, poorer self-judgment, and susceptibility to denial and avoidance during a time of illness (Abend, 1982; Dewald, 1982; Schwartz, 1987; Laskey, 1990). Arlow (1990) wrote about the defensive distortions that could occur in one's perception at a time of illness, using his experience during and after a series of heart attacks. He was struck "by how strong was my need to deny the gravity of my illness and how this tendency was buttressed by my adopting an 'analytic' attitude of participant observer" (p. 19). He concluded that whatever one decided to disclose or not disclose would be determined by both conscious and unconscious motives.

Prior to the 1990s, many analysts (Abend, 1982; Dewald, 1982; Schwartz, 1987; Laskey, 1990) recommended against disclosure. Primarily, this was to not overburden the patient with one's illness and to preserve a safe, neutral space in which a patient's transferences could most optimally unfold and be interpreted. Dewald (1982) believed that an analyst who disclosed his illness would be tempted to react defensively and promote premature closure of more threatening affect rather than explore the full gamut of the patient's emotions and associations to the illness. Over time, there has been a broadening perspective on whether to disclose factual information about one's illness and the impact of such disclosure or nondisclosure. During this same time there have also been more reports by women analysts about their experiences with illness and cancer, often breast cancer, and its impact on clinical work with patients (Silver, 1982, 1990, 2001; Morrison, 1990, 1997; Friedman, 1991; Clark, 1995; Pizer, 1997; Schwaber, 1998; Fajardo, 2001; Kahn, 2003). Many of these same reports have also stressed the positive and mobilizing effect of disclosure on the therapeutic relationship and treatment (Silver, 1992, 2001; Pizer, 1997; Schwaber, 1998; Fajardo, 2001; Kahn, 2003).

Even those analysts recommending nondisclosure have reported that they often could not put into practice what they recommended (Abend, 1982; Dewald, 1982; Friedman, 1991). Patients would hear about their illnesses from other sources (Dewald, 1982); analysts would underestimate how long their recovery would take (Schwartz, 1987); and changes in their physical appearance made it more difficult to treat patients' reactions only as a fantasy (Abend, 1982). Therefore, a reading of the analytic literature suggests to me that analysts, depending on their circumstances and those of their patients, had to adapt to the reality of their circumstances and do what they judged would best allow the analytic work to go forth. Halpert (1982) describes the destructive results to patients whose analysts did not adapt. Their analysts were in denial and did not disclose their illness nor prepare their patients for their impending death. In contrast, Feinsilver (1998), who had metastatic colon cancer and was dying, disclosed his medical condition to his patients because he wanted them to be aware how the reality of his illness would affect their work, including the option to find a new therapist. Feinsilver believed that the awareness of death had a limit-setting and mobilizing effect on his work with patients.

PERSONAL BACKGROUND

At the time I learned about my breast cancer, I was both in analysis and in supervision with three different supervisors. I had the personal support of my family and friends, including two fellow candidate/classmates who were breast cancer survivors. As a result, I believe I had significantly more support than most therapists confronted by a life-threatening diagnosis. I believe this was critical in my being able to work more comfortably with my patients. It was also reassuring to learn, after my surgery, that the cancer had not progressed into my lymph nodes. I recovered quickly after my lumpectomy. Physically, the most difficult time for me was after my chemotherapy treatments, when I was more fatigued and nauseous. I was able to manage this with more rest and by scheduling my chemotherapy treatments on a Friday, with almost three days to recover. I experienced working during my cancer treatment as actually helpful to me. It focused me on understanding my patients' concerns and reinforced my need to feel competent and capable.

The most difficult emotional time that I had with my cancer was at the beginning when I knew the least about it, was frightened, and was undergoing further biopsies and tests and interviewing surgeons. I could hardly imagine telling my patients about my cancer. I thought it would be crushing and overwhelming to them, no doubt similar to how I first felt about it. When I informed my supervisors about having cancer and sought their advice about how to handle this with my patients, my disclosure spurred greater exposure and expressions of support on their part. All of my supervisors shared with me something personal about their own personal and family experiences with health-related matters, including cancer. My supervisors differed in their recommendations as to how to handle my cancer with patients. Two of my supervisors encouraged me to directly and openly bring up my cancer diagnosis with my patients, as they believed that it was something that could not be hidden and that my patients would unconsciously know that something was different. My other supervisor recommended a more measured approach, based upon my patient's readiness as revealed by her associations in the session. Another analyst suggested that I needed to think about my own needs and feelings in deciding what I would reveal to my patients. My own analyst suggested I might want to read a paper by Evelyn Schwaber (1998). It was "'Traveling Affectively Alone': A Personal Derailment in Analytic Listening," in which Schwaber spoke about her personal experience with breast cancer and what allowed her to become more emotionally engaged and attuned to her patients.

I decided to tell all my patients that I would need to take off one-and-a-half weeks of work in order to attend to some personal health matters (it was my surgeon who recommended that I take off ten days post-surgery). I made this announcement as soon as I received a firm date for my lumpectomy. My surgery was three weeks from the day I first received my cancer diagnosis. I had roughly a week to inform my patients and work with their reactions to my taking time off. I decided I would disclose more if their response and subsequent associations indicated they needed to know more. I wanted to explore their fantasies about my absence, but I also felt a need for some measure of honesty in my response. I did not have this well thought out in the weeks before my surgery. I was aware that some level of disclosure would help me to be more emotionally engaged with my patients, hear their reactions and fantasies to my health crisis, and analyze and interpret more freely. Ultimately, my analytic patients and most of my psychotherapy patients learned that I was having surgery for a malignant breast tumor that had been found early.

There were a few patients with whom I did not disclose my cancer. Typically, they were newer patients with whom I met with once a week or less frequently, and I had thought our meeting schedule would not be much interrupted by upcoming chemotherapy and radiation appointments. Interestingly, but not too surprisingly, the psychotherapy patients whom I did not disclose the reasons for my health break broke off treatment in the ten months following my surgery. This did not happen with patients with whom I disclosed my cancer condition. While there are numerous factors contributing to this, I think, for the most part, this happened because these patients sensed that something had happened with me but did not feel they could bring it up. Possibly, some felt a sense of betrayal because I had not told them. All of my patients, I believe, experienced anxiety and anger at me for "getting sick" and potentially abandoning them, but there was more opportunity to point this out and work with it therapeutically when the elephant in the room (my health condition) could be talked about, tolerated, and understood.

I would not have been able to work with patients had I not had a private place of my own in which to voice, discover, and understand my own feelings and reactions to my cancer diagnosis. Fantasies and fears of dying were most palpable even as I tried to be as proactive as I could in understanding my cancer and interviewing surgeons and oncologists. The learning curve was steep, but I threw myself into it. I learned early on, and throughout the subsequent months, that many women have had breast cancer during their lifetime. Many were willing to talk about it upon learning I had cancer and was in need of advice about doctors, treatment, what to expect, etc. Over time, especially as I wrote about my cancer experience, I discovered many professional colleagues who had also dealt with cancer but had not revealed it to colleagues and patients, frequently out of fear that they would lose patients and referrals, or that revealing a cancer condition would be too much exposure for them or for their patients to bear.

For myself, I found it very informative and helpful to become aware of the sisterhood of breast cancer survivors. For example, I experienced great support when one of my professional colleagues, a breast cancer survivor herself, offered to accompany me when I went shopping for a wig. The anticipation of losing my long hair as a result of chemotherapy was more difficult than I had expected. I think this was because my hair was such a tangible symbol of all that I was losing—not only my hair and familiar appearance, but also my sense of security, and possibly, my life. In a proactive move, I had my head shaved prior to losing my hair. This was both practical and yet another way of lessening feelings of helplessness by making a decision that I controlled. The emotional support I received from my colleague who was present with me as my head was being shaved was enormous. Moments before I was able to turn around and look at myself in a mirror, she said to me: "You know, you really do have a nice-shaped head." These words stay with me still because her presence and empathic comment made it easier for me to face what I feared I would see—someone different from the "me" I had known. In hindsight, I think her comment helped dispel a preconscious, fear-filled fantasy—that of looking unattractive, bald, and deathly skull-like without my hair.

MY ANALYSIS

My analyst, of course, did not accompany me to wig appointments, but she did accompany me in very emotionally attuned, analytic ways so that I felt and was less alone. While I was fortunate to have had good family, friends, doctors, colleagues, and breast cancer survivors who supported me during my cancer treatment, there are some things that are difficult to talk about and for others to hear. There are limitations in such otherwise valuable relationships, especially if you are a working professional with patients or clients. Many want to help and do help in significant ways, but they are not accustomed to or may be afraid of intense feelings and thoughts that could surface in you or in them. I have experienced and seen other cancer patients be told or encouraged to feel "positive," "hopeful," and "optimistic," while going through cancer treatment. While hope is a good and necessary ingredient for most undertakings in life, there are many, including health providers, who undervalue the importance of listening, tolerating, bearing, and understanding a patient's worst fears and nightmares about cancer, especially thoughts of death. Frequently, I came across others telling me to "not dwell on it," or "don't go there" (*there* being thoughts of dying). The fear and belief behind these admonitions is that if one thinks and verbalizes such "bad or negative thoughts" (that is, thoughts about suffering, relapsing, and dying), that this type of thinking could *actually* make one's condition worse.

In other words, many loved ones worry that if you are not positive but feel negative, that this, in itself, could fuel cancer cell growth or weaken your immune system's ability to "fight" the cancer. This is one area where my analysis and analyst was most helpful. My analyst would remind me of what I knew but needed to hear—that voicing my fears and thinking about dying would not fuel cancer growth, would not hurt me, and that it was better to air these thoughts and think about and understand them. At the same time, while she would listen to my fears and sadness, she would also acknowledge where she thought I was being overly pessimistic or ill-informed. I remember, early on, to her listening to my fears, acknowledging them but also reminding me that "even if the cancer has spread into your lymph nodes, that that is not fatal. There can be successful treatment of that." Her hope was present in various ways. For example, she strongly encouraged that I take good notes of my work with patients because they would be valuable to write up at some point. It would make for a good paper and a valuable contribution to our profession. By envisioning a future for me beyond or with cancer, she helped me to find meaning in all that I was going through, and to keep hope alive that I could actualize that vision.

I remember a dream that I brought into my analysis around the time of my lumpectomy surgery. I did not understand, initially, its connection to current fears. In the dream, I was at the side entrance of my childhood home, at the door that I most typically entered when I was a child. Something looked different about the door. There was something in the corner of the door that I couldn't quite see. There was something about the corner that was different. My associations, at first, seemed sparse and opaque, but my analyst asked me to continue to associate to "corner." Then, it hit me. I was surprised—it might have been the way she emphasized or pronounced the word, but I thought of "coroner." This reference to death led me to my fears about dying. Other associations to my childhood house, which was made of brick, and which we moved into when I was three, reminded me of a familiar story from childhood—that of "The Three Little Pigs." The story tells of the three different houses that each of the three pigs built—one of straw, one of wood, and one of bricks—to protect them from the clutches of the big, bad wolf who wanted to kill and eat them. Which house would best withstand the huffs and puffs of the big bad wolf? The one built of bricks. The understanding (and interpretation) that came from this dream was my wish and hope that my house, my body, would be strong and sturdy enough to withstand cancer and death and the upcoming chemo and radiation treatments. My actual childhood house was made of bricks, and I hoped my early home/life structure would provide me the strength I needed at this time of duress.

There is no doubt that at the time of my cancer diagnosis and subsequent treatment for it that I was afraid of dying. I learned to tolerate and talk about these fears. The most difficult time was at the beginning when I knew the least about my cancer. The most terrible fantasies and deepest emotions preoccupied me. I found myself thinking about an attractive, educated, articulate woman whom I had known in our neighborhood several years earlier. I had seen her journey from health and vibrancy to a frail, emaciated, hairless image of her former self, despite multiple treatments and her prayers for remission of her breast cancer, and, eventually, to her death. I worried that her fate could be mine. As I gained more information about the different types of breast cancer, I learned that she had suffered from inflammatory breast cancer—a most lethal type—but a type different from my own. Becoming more informed was helpful to me, as was airing all these fears in my own treatment. I was further relieved, following my lumpectomy, to learn that my lymph nodes were cancer free, that margins were good, and that it was a stage I cancer. Because of the type of cancer I had, for which estrogen-suppressing drugs were not an effective deterrent to prevent a reoccurrence, chemotherapy and radiation were recommended. The idea was to attack and destroy, early on, as many cancer cells that might still be present. Facing chemotherapy and radiation, while daunting for me, was less psychologically fearful because it represented an actual, active form of fighting cancer. I was "doing something" that would be helping me, even while unpleasant. I believed my house of bricks could withstand it.

My analysis, certainly, was very helpful. But was my analysis different during the time of my cancer treatment? Did my analyst treat me differently during this time? I have been asked these questions by others, I believe, in an attempt to differentiate what is helpful in the treatment of patients facing life-threatening illnesses as well as to understand the benefits of an analytic perspective at such times. I believe a major benefit is to have an analyst who can tolerate intense and frightening feelings and fantasies, not closing them off but allowing them to come fully into the room to be contained, verbalized, explored, understood, and integrated into one's ego. Even when there are fears not yet understood, there is an immense value in being heard, accompanied, and held in the mind of your therapist. In most ways, my analyst did not behave differently during my cancer treatment and after it than at other times. However, I felt her presence more. She seemed less in the background and more interactive, but that also might have been my need to feel her closer to me. More likely, it was both. Her interest and concern were clearly felt when she would ask me to let her know how a particular test or procedure went—be it by phone or e-mail—rather than to just wait until my session time. These communications were very brief. We talked and analyzed in the session, not in the e-mail or voicemail, although she would always respond to my communication in a few words, or just "Thanks." I felt accompanied.

During the time of my cancer treatment, I continued to use the couch, and the analysis proceeded along psychoanalytic lines, although what I most frequently dealt with in my sessions were my reactions and fears about cancer and about my work with patients. My analyst considered it part of her job to not only help me with my unconscious but also with current reality intrusions (recognizing that these were also influenced by my fantasies). I had chosen to work with my analyst prior to beginning analytic training. She encouraged and supported my decision to begin analytic training at which time she became my training analyst. I have always experienced her as caring and a very good listener.

The idea of being accompanied, heard, not alone has been an important theme throughout my cancer treatment. It relates strongly to my anxieties about dying. I found a certain psalm spontaneously coming to mind numerous times during my daytime and nighttime thoughts and reflections. It was later that I learned it was from Psalm 23: "Yea, though I walk through the valley of the shadow of death, I will fear no evil: For Thou art with me, at my side." I did fear, but I was learning to tolerate this fear. The psalm brought comfort and reflected both my anxiety about death and my wish to be accompanied on this journey, which I hoped would not be a final one.

CLINICAL WORK

How did my cancer and my disclosure of it affect my patients and their treatment? For my patients in analysis, and from the perspective of more than five years from first diagnosis, these analyses progressed and deepened, as judged by the patients, by me, and by my Institute supervisors (I graduated nineteen months from the time I was diagnosed with cancer). I do not know how my work with them would have been different had I not had cancer or not disclosed it. As for my psychotherapy patients, their therapies continued to deepen and progress, especially if there was an established therapeutic alliance prior to my cancer.

All of my patients to whom I disclosed my cancer condition responded in some ways similarly: they feared losing me to death; they worried what would happen to them and their treatments; they hoped that I had sufficient supports outside the treatment; they wanted to be helpful to me; and they struggled with how much they could tell me about their needs and feelings, especially anger, at a time of greater perceived and actual vulnerability for me. Disclosure of my cancer evoked for them countless memories of other illnesses and losses of people in their lives. It also evoked anxiety and fantasies about "seeing" more about me. On the other hand, the few psychotherapy patients whom I did not disclose my cancer broke off treatment in the ten months following my surgery. This did not happen with patients whom I disclosed my cancer condition. I described earlier in this chapter my understanding of why this might have happened. I had not told some of these patients because I was not meeting as frequently or regularly with them, and thought my cancer treatment schedule would not impact my session times with them. In another case, I did not inform a once-a-week patient because she had just lost her husband after many months of seeing him progressively and painfully decline in health. Consciously, I wanted to spare her further worry. She mourned his death, but stopped treatment shortly after I began chemotherapy and told me she was doing better and could manage on her own. She was doing better, but I think there was much we could not address.

In retrospect, my cancer posed a real-life threat to me and my patients and their therapies, as well as eliciting multiple fantasies along transference lines. It was a real-life event that became interwoven with their personal histories and fantasies. It heightened my patients' awareness of transference feelings, their relationship to me, and my importance to them. I believe that my measured disclosure of my cancer enhanced the therapeutic alliance with patients. Without my own analysis and supervision, it would not have been as possible to effectively continue working with my patients. I would not have been able to hear and tolerate my patients' fears that I could die, nor would I have been as able to work with their anger at me for burdening their treatment with my illness unless I could tolerate my own feelings and fears of death. I will share some clinical vignettes from my analytic practice which highlight the meanings and impact of my cancer and its disclosure on my patients. Greater clinical elaboration and discussion is to be found in an earlier paper (Plopa, 2009).

Case 1

Susan was a perceptive, vigilant, creative woman with a background of trauma and depression. She began our first session after my lumpectomy surgery by telling me that she suspected from the onset that my medical health break was due to cancer, even though she had not said this previously. When I first told Susan that I would be taking time off for health procedures, she asked no questions. However, in subsequent material, she related how frustrating and difficult it was in her family when parents kept secrets and never informed the children about their health problems, causing the children to worry and be frightened. Five months earlier, Susan's mother informed her that she would be having surgery—for stomach cancer. This was devastating to Susan, but not completely a surprise. Her mother had never said anything about consulting doctors and undergoing medical tests. Yet, three months before her mother's announcement, Susan had noticed and worried that her mother was looking thinner and more forlorn. However, Susan had learned not to inquire about these matters. Susan herself had undergone many medical procedures in early childhood, which were traumatic for her and contributed to her vigilance.

"I knew it. The moment you first said about taking time off, I knew it was breast cancer." I asked her how she knew. Susan responded: "You looked fine. Cancer is invisible, especially early on. It's sinister. And it happens a lot. You know, I think I had some feeling about it even before you told me about taking time off." Susan proceeded to tell me that she had reviewed what she had written in her personal journal. She read to me the entry for a date in September, which was before the date I learned about my cancer diagnosis. Susan had written: "Dr. P. seems more subdued today, quieter, maybe sad. I wonder if there is something wrong. I hope it is nothing really serious." I asked her to tell me the date for this entry. The day she wrote this was shortly after our session and the day before my breast biopsy. I had thought I was focused on my patient during that session. But my patient was sensitive to something that seemed different about me, even though I was not aware of coming across differently in the session. Interestingly, in my notes for that same session, I had also noted that Susan seemed "quieter" and "more subdued."

In subsequent sessions, Susan joked about how I was making things difficult for her because I was adding confusion to her mother transference to me. She had to keep reminding herself that my cancer was much more treatable and curable than her mother's cancer. Her mother was going through chemotherapy and radiation treatments. Susan made herself very available to help out her mother. Susan wanted to be helpful to me, a part of my "healing team." Disclosing my cancer to Susan initially promoted feelings and fantasies of inclusion. However, I did not tell Susan when I was beginning my chemotherapy as I did not see a need for this. In addition, I believed it would become apparent to her that I was having chemotherapy when I began to wear a wig. Nondisclosure of my chemotherapy treatments brought up intense feelings of exclusion, rejection, and anger which also resonated with childhood experiences. Acknowledging and working through these feelings over time helped Susan to become less afraid that her anger and rage could hurt or kill me. Working through this fear that her rage could destroy the relationships she most depended on continued well beyond my return to health and the death of her own mother from cancer. So fearful was Susan about losing me that for a long time she, who was typically so vigilant, continued to believe that I had not lost my hair and that my wig was my real hair. Susan had witnessed her mother's progressive decline and ultimate death, and she feared seeing signs (wearing a wig) that I would decline and die.

Case 2

The disclosure of my cancer to John, a depressed, middle-age, divorced man who tended to minimize feelings, connections, and reactions to me and to significant others, had the effect of making the transference much more noticeable, palpable, and analyzable. The impact of my cancer surfaced in associations, dreams, and recollections and made an impression that helped him recognize the depth of his feelings toward me. He also came closer to recognizing the ways in which he had distanced himself from his mother and from mourning her recent death.

Shortly after we started the analysis, John's mother died from advanced cancer, which John knew little about because he had avoided contact with her. John's reaction to her death was intellectualized and philosophical, and he insisted that he had mourned her tragic life years before. John initially asked few questions when I announced my break, but there were subsequent associations to a female friend who was dying of cancer. I suggested he might also be concerned about my health. He inquired about my health, asking if the cancer was life-threatening. He said that his mother had been riddled with cancer when she died and had never taken care of herself. I told John that I was having a lumpectomy at an early stage of cancer and addressed his worries about whether I would be able to care for myself, unlike his mother who had not been able to care adequately for herself or for him. In the next session, John discussed an article he read about the dangers of multitasking. I responded by telling him that I thought he was worried about whether I could focus on him and his concerns at the same time I was dealing with cancer. John hoped I would have people able to help me as I went through treatment.

The disclosure of my cancer intensified feelings in the therapy relationship and transference. Following my surgery and over the next seven months, during my chemotherapy and radiation treatment, John related many incidents and stories about women who were dealing with illness, cancer, or had died. He worried about a friend who had been in a bad accident and was amazed that he prayed for her. This was striking to him because he did not believe in prayer or a personal God. He began to visit a dying elderly woman in a nursing home. He was surprised that the experience was gratifying to him as well as to her. John contrasted his involvement with her to how he had stayed distant from his mother. "Being with this woman has made me aware of not being there with my mother." Discussion of his avoidance of his mother led to a greater awareness of how he had long felt abandoned by his mother because of her self-absorption and problems. I added that he worried that I might leave him on his own before he was able to work issues out for himself. John could not address directly, for some time, any anger that he felt toward me for adding this extra issue to his analysis.

DISCUSSION AND CONCLUSION

There are two factors that I believe were critical and helped me immensely in working with my patients during the time of my cancer diagnosis and treatment. The first is that I did not die, become incapacitated, or appear very ill. Even when feeling ill (tired or nauseated), I continued—in a "good-enough" way—to be able to listen, understand, and withstand their biggest fears—that I would die, leave them, or be unable to help them with their feelings. Had I fared worse, their treatments might have struggled more.

> As it was, all of my patients had intense fears about my possible demise. They worried about my vulnerability—as a patient and as a candidate-analyst. What facilitated the identification and working through of their fantasies about losing me or hurting me was the reality that I did not die and that I remained in empathic contact with them. I stayed and worked with them and I got better.

Whatever destructive fantasies they feared in themselves in connection with
my cancer were made weaker by my continuing to work and live. (Plopa,
2009, p. 29)

The disclosure of my cancer to patients—a measured, selective disclosure—
actually, in hindsight, seemed to build trust and enhance the therapeutic
alliance. To name the elephant in the room (my cancer) and to talk about
what that meant to my patients gave me a greater sense of freedom and
personal workspace to emotionally engage with my patients, hear associations, and analyze.

The second factor of major significance was that I was not alone. I had
family, friends, professional colleagues, a good medical team, and the help
and support of my supervisors, especially my analyst. My patients were
concerned that I have ample supports and resources for myself, not only
because they wished me well but also to allay their fears of having to take
care of me. Believing I had such resources helped to allay fears that their
feelings could hurt me and burden me. I would not have felt as focused and
able to tolerate patients' feelings and fears had I not had places where I could
address and sort through my needs and fears and those of my patients. Consequently, I believe that making good clinical judgments and working effectively at a time of illness is both possible and enhanced by outside consultation, professional support, and one's own analytic treatment (Plopa, 2009).

In conclusion, what have I learned about the treatment of cancer patients
from my own experience of being a cancer patient, and now, in subsequent
years, from my treatment of cancer patients in my own practice and from
volunteer work that I do at local hospitals with cancer patients? It is this: the
importance of hearing patients' stories and staying affectively connected
with them. This involves affect tolerance and the ability to mourn while
staying affectively connected to loving others. We aim to accompany our
patients, holding in mind their past identities and values, hearing and holding
their present fears and wishes, helping them tolerate and verbalize their current fears, feelings, and hopes, and promoting their ability to visualize a
meaningful future, even if that means confronting and thinking about death.

Many years ago, as a young psychologist, I participated in a study group
with psychoanalyst Richard Sterba not many years before he died. Richard
Sterba was in the first graduating class of the Vienna Psychoanalytic Institute
and emigrated to the United States in 1939. It was a fascinating study group
and Dr. Sterba relished telling us young therapists stories about psychoanalysis and psychoanalysts in the "early days." The only quote from Sterba that I
never forgot was one that he attributed to Freud shortly before Freud died.
Freud was in great pain at this point and dying from cancer. According to
Sterba, Freud told his physician: "I am on an island of pain in the midst of a
sea of indifference" (Sterba, 1987). I never saw references to this quote until

I was reading Schur (1972, p. 724), who noted a similar passage from Freud to Marie Bonaparte in a letter dated June 16, 1939. The quote from Sterba about Freud had struck me at the first time I heard it, and through the subsequent years, as so sad and so lonely and so dark. I believe I never forgot this line because it caused me to reflect on the loneliness of death and the helplessness we feel in the immediate face of it. Freud, however, in so many ways, was not alone in that he had a devoted physician and many devoted followers who cared deeply about him. His body was also under very painful attack from his cancer. Nevertheless, Paul of Tarsus (1 Corinthians 15: 26–27) may have had it right: Death is the last enemy we all have to face. And we experience it alone. But for patients we treat and who are still with us—we accompany them.

REFERENCES

Abend, S. (1982). Serious illness in the analyst: Countertransference considerations. *Journal of the American Psychoanalytic Association, 30*, 365–379.

Arlow, J. (1990). The analytic attitude in the service of denial. In H. J. Schwartz & A.-L. Silver (Eds.), *Illness in the Analyst* (pp. 9–26). Madison, CT: International Universities Press, 1992.

Clark, R. (1995). The Pope's confessor: A metaphor relating to illness in the analyst. *Journal of the American Psychoanalytic Association, 43*, 137–149.

Dewald, P. A. (1982). Serious illness in the analyst: Transference, countertransference, and reality responses. *Journal of American Psychoanalytic Association, 30*, 347–363.

Fajardo, B. (2001). Life-threatening illness in the analyst. *Journal of the American Psychoanalytic Association, 49*, 569–586.

Feinsilver, D. B. (1998). The therapist as a person facing death: The hardest of external realities and therapeutic action. *International Journal of Psychoanalysis, 79*, 1131–1150.

Fieldsteel, N. D. (1989). Analysts' expressed attitudes toward dealing with death and illness. *Contemporary Psychoanalysis, 25*, 427–43.

Friedman, G. (1991). Impact of a therapist's life threatening illness on the therapeutic situation. *Contemporary Psychoanalysis, 27*, 405–421.

Halpert, E. (1982). When the analyst is chronically ill or dying. *Psychoanalytic Quarterly, 51*, 372–389.

Kahn, N. E. (2003). Self-disclosure of serious illness: The impact of boundary disruptions for patient and analyst. *Contemporary Psychoanalysis, 39*, 51–74.

Laskey, R. (1990). Catastrophic illness in the analyst and the analyst's emotional reactions to it. *International Journal of Psychoanalysis, 71*, 455–473.

Morrison, A. L. (1990). Doing psychotherapy while living with a life-threatening illness. In H. J. Schwartz & A.-L. Silver (Eds.), *Illness in the Analyst* (pp. 227–250). Madison, CT: International Universities Press.

———. (1997). Ten years of doing psychotherapy while living with a life-threatening illness: Self-disclosure and other ramifications. *Psychoanalytic Dialogue, 7*, 225–241.

Pizer, B. (1997). When the analyst is ill: Dimensions of self-disclosure. *The Psychoanalytic Quarterly, 66*, 450–469.

Plopa, P. (2009). Cancer, candidacy, and the couch. Unpublished paper. Awarded 2009 scientific paper prize by Affiliate Council. Presented at January 2010 APsaA meeting.

Schur, M. (1972). *Freud: Living and dying*. New York: International Universities Press.

Schwaber, E. A. (1998). "Traveling affectively alone": A personal derailment in analytic listening. *Journal of the American Psychoanalytic Association, 46*, 1045–1065.

Schwartz, H. J. (1987). Illness in the doctor: Implications for psychoanalytic process. *Journal of the American Psychoanalytic Association, 35*, 657–692.

Schwartz, H. J., & Silver, A.-L. (Eds.). (1990). *Illness in the analyst: Implications for the treatment relationship.* Madison, CT: International Universities Press.

Silver, A-L. (1982). Resuming the work with a life-threatening illness. *Contemporary Psychoanalysis, 18*, 314–326.

———. (1990). Resuming the work with a life threatening illness—and further reflections. In H. J. Schwartz & A.-L. Silver (Eds.), *Illness in the Analyst* (pp. 151–176). Madison, CT: International Universities Press.

———. (2001). Facing mortality while treating patients: A plea for a measure of authenticity. *Journal of the American Academy of Psychoanalysis, 29*, 43–56.

Conclusion

Norman Straker, MD

The main goal of this book has been to recognize the important role that "death anxiety" plays in all aspects of health care. This required a review of where we are now and why and what remedies might be considered. I began by illustrating how quickly any public discussion of funding for counseling for end-of-life care was dropped because of how easily it can be manipulated for political gain (for example, the Obama death panels). Attempts at discourse about the end-of-life medical treatment almost immediately evoke the fear that saving money will take priority over saving lives. We need to recognize that many of our citizens fear that any policy changes will give those in authority the ability to abuse it to save money.

This same underlying mistrust was manifest in the case of the patient whose medical treatment cost over $2.1 million in one year, as reported in a review article in the *Wall Street Journal* (chapter 1). When the doctor approached the patient's father, on several occasions, about discussing future treatment goals for his son, the father accused the doctor of wanting permission to let his son die to save the hospital money. At that time, the son was unable to speak, appeared to be terminally ill, and was suffering with no hope of cure. The doctor denied that accusation but seemed to be so off guard and defensive that he was unable to firmly state why end-of-life care would be preferable to futile care or ask for a mental health consult. This interchange suggests that powerful unconscious forces were present in both the father and the doctor. Unfortunately, no mental health professional was called to try to work through the conflict.

This encounter suggests that the doctor and the father had a great need to defend against their unconscious murderous impulses. The father displaced his murderous impulses onto the doctor, accusing him of wanting permission to end the life of his son. The doctor defensively denied the accusation as if it was a rational accusation and continued the futile treatments as if to prove that the accusation had no merit. It is hard to know how commonly this dynamic is a part of the motivation for futile treatments, but it is certainly worth further study.

A central hypothesis in the book has been that end-of-life care discussions are often avoided and delayed because of collusion between doctors, patients, and families who defend against death anxiety. The fact that one-third of the Medicare budget is spent in the last year of patient's life reflects this unresolved problem. At the same time, I have documented through both published studies and case reports, that oncologists who do not cope effectively with death anxiety and grief are prone to dissociation, suppression, and excessive drinking, which can lead to mental complicated grief, depression, PTSD, burnout, and so forth.

I have suggested some remedies for these problems. I have recommended that our medical culture be changed so that medical students and doctors can learn the importance of accepting and processing the emotional impact of facing life-and-death decisions. This will allow them to become more mindful of their emotional conflicts and how their state of mind can affect medical decisions. I have also suggested group support and debriefing of oncology, psycho-oncology fellows, and residents after a death of their patient to prevent dissociation and numbing that can lead to avoidance and, eventually, burnout.

As we doctors realize the complexity of the decision-making process that leads to recommending the end of active treatment and starting palliative care it becomes apparent that it would be less burdensome to the individual doctor if this became a shared decision. Perhaps, after some established objective criterion is reached for a patient that defines terminal illness (to be determined) it would trigger a committee of peers (ethics committee?) to review future treatment goals. Such a committee would decrease the emotional burden on the individual physician and would support a discussion with the patient and family on the current medical facts, treatment options, and prognosis. If the patient, family, and doctor cannot agree on what seems to be a rational plan for palliation, a meeting with a mental health professional would be a next step. The task for the mental health professional would be to mediate the conflict by uncovering the individual conflicts that have stalled an acceptance of the inevitable. The mental health professional needs to be someone who understands unconscious conflicts and is comfortable with confrontation and resolution of these issues. If this meeting is unsuccessful, a recommendation for further exploration could be made with a therapist.

The second major goal of this book was to help psychoanalysts become more at ease with the concept of death anxiety, facing death, treating dying patients, and, finally, recruiting them to bring their knowledge of unconscious conflict to the hospital where they can help their medical colleagues with the complexity of end-of-life issues. A review of the literature and multiple case reports have been presented to encourage psychoanalysts to feel more at ease with treating dying patients in a flexible but uniquely psychoanalytic manner. While some in the past have written about maintaining an orthodox technique, their recommendation is based on single case descriptions. They fail to accept the view that facing death is a very unique experience, unlike suffering from neurosis and character issues that require maintaining the basic concepts of psychoanalytic treatment modified to fit a unique situation. To that point, I have made some recommendations for end-of-life psychoanalytic treatment that are practical, relevant, and meaningful to a population of patients facing death. These recommendations are based on more than thirty-five years of work with cancer patients, supervision, and yearly analytic case discussions at the American Psychoanalytic Association meetings.

If death anxiety is confronted more directly and made less frightening, patients, the families of the patients, medical professionals, and society in general would all benefit greatly. For patients, there would be less suffering, and they would be not subject to cruel treatment that continues unnecessarily. For families of patients, there would be less guilt and possibly even the realization or satisfaction that the family had acted with greater compassion and love. For the medical professional, there would also be less survivor guilt, dissociation, PTSD, depression, and complicated grief. Finally, for society there would be an improved health care system and a more rational allocation of limited financial and medical resources.

REFERENCE

Adamy, J., & McGinty, T. (2012, July 7–9). The crushing cost of medical care. *Wall Street Journal*, online.wsj.com.

Index

ABDT. *See* anxiety buffer disruption theory
Adams-Silvan, A., 65, 83–100, 155
advance directives, 5; prevalence and predictors of, 5
AMA. *See* American Medical Association
American Medical Association (AMA), x
anaphylaxis, 28
antidepressants, 95
antithymocyte globulin (ATG), 27–28
anxiety: about death, ix, xi; of physicians, 17; terminal diagnosis and, 52. *See also* case examples
anxiety buffer disruption theory (ABDT), 46–48
ATG (antithymocyte globulin), 27–28
attachment theory, 66

Bail, B., 64
Barnhill, John W., 103–113, 155
Becker, Ernest, 33, 43
Berzoff, J., 65
Birger, Daniel, 23–24, 26–32, 156
Breitbart, William, 24, 56, 67
Buprioprion, for treatment of depression, 10
Bustamante, J. J., 65

cancer: cost of care, 147, 149; denial of, 22, 69; diagnosis of, 21–22; disclosure versus nondisclosure, 133–135; hospital culture and, 8–9; literature, 133–134; outpatient treatment for, 108; pain management, 73; patient distress prior to treatment for, 54; patient in analysis while working as an analyst, 131–145; phobia of, 23–24; psychotherapy for a middle-aged woman with, 83–100; recurrence of, 21–22; remission of, 86; "sisterhood" of survivors, 136; survival of, 24; treatment of, 18, 63, 69–79. *See also* case examples; hospice; palliative care
case examples, x–xi; of a cancer patient in analysis while working as an analyst, 131–145; of death anxiety and demoralization, 76–78; end of life, 15–17; lack of, xi; of patient survival time issues, 71–73; of psychotherapy of a middle-aged woman with cancer, 83–100; of psychotherapy of a young woman with cancer, 103–113; of psychotherapy with a hospitalized patient dying of cancer, 123–129; of recommended principles for flexible psychoanalytic psychotherapy for cancer patients, 115–121
Christian Science, 93
CL. *See* consultation-liaison service
clergy, counseling patients, 22
communication, xi; outcomes from talking about death, 6

151

About the Contributors

Norman Straker, MD, edited this book and offered an approach for facing death and the treatment of cancer patients based on thirty-five years of clinical experience. Dr. Straker was one of the original faculty members of the very first psycho-oncology services under the leadership of Dr. Jimmie Holland at Memorial Sloan-Kettering Cancer Center. He remains active there today in teaching and research. He is also a clinical professor of psychiatry at Weill Cornell College of Medicine and teaches residents in psychiatry, oncology, and palliative care at the Mount Sinai Medical Center. He is a psychoanalyst and a member of the faculty of the New York Psychoanalytic Institute where he also teaches courses on psychoanalytic psychotherapy of cancer patients. He has chaired a discussion group, "Psychoanalysis and Psychoanalytic Psychotherapy of Cancer Patients," at the American Psychoanalytic Association for more than twenty-five years. He is in private practice in New York City.

ABOUT THE CONTRIBUTORS

Abby Adams-Silvan, PhD, is a training analyst, faculty member, and a past president of the Contemporary New York Freudian Society. She is also an associate clinical professor at the New York University Postdoctoral Program in Psychoanalysis and Psychotherapy. She is in private practice.

John W. Barnhill, MD, is professor of clinical psychiatry and vice chair for psychosomatic medicine at the Weill Cornell Medical College. He is also chief of consultation-liaison psychiatry at the New York Presbyterian Hospital/Weill Cornell Medical Center. He serves on the faculty at the Columbia Psychoanalytic Center.

Daniel Birger, MD, is assistant clinical professor at the Mout Sinai School of Medicine, New York. He is on the faculty of the New York Psychoanalytic Institute. He is also in private practice.

M. Philip Luber, MD, is associate professor of psychiatry and director of Education and Residency Training at the University of Maryland Medical Center. He is also a graduate of the New York Psychoanalytic Institute.

Molly Maxfield, PhD, is assistant professor of psychology and director of the Undergraduate Honors Program at the University of Colorado, Colorado Springs.

Alison C. Phillips, MD, is an advanced candidate at the Boston Psychoanalytic Society. She is in private practice.

Patricia Plopa, PhD, is adjunct professor of the clinical psychology graduate program at the University of Detroit, Mercy. She is president-elect of the Michigan Psychoanalytic Society, where she is also on the faculty. She is in private practice.

Tom Pyszczynski, PhD, is distinguished professor of psychology at the University of Colorado, Colorado Springs.

Sheldon Solomon, PhD, is professor of social psychology at Skidmore College.

Hillel Swiller, MD, is clinical professor of psychiatry and chief of the Psychotherapy Department at the Mount Sinai School of Medicine, New York. He is a graduate of the New York Psychoanalytic Institute and is also in private practice.

David P. Yuppa, MD, is attending psychiatrist at the Dana-Farber Cancer Institute, associate psychiatrist at the Brigham and Women's Hospital, and an instructor of psychiatry at Harvard Medical School.

Made in the USA
Middletown, DE
07 December 2016